AF327200

Hypertension Therapy Annual

Hypertension Therapy Annual

Edited by

Norman M Kaplan MD

Professor of Internal Medicine
University of Texas Southwestern Medical Center
Dallas TX

Martin Dunitz

First published in the United Kingdom in 2000 by
Martin Dunitz Ltd
The Livery House
7–9 Pratt Street
London NW1 0AE

Tel: +44-(0)20-7482-2202
Fax: +44-(0)20-7267-0159
E-mail: info@mdunitz.globalnet.co.uk
Website: http://www.dunitz.co.uk

A CIP catalogue record for this book is available from the British Library

ISBN 1-85317-728-8

Distributed in the United States by:
Blackwell Science Inc.
Commerce Place, 350 Main Street
Malden MA 02148, USA
Tel: 1-800-215-1000

Distributed in Canada by:
Login Brothers Book Company
324 Salteaux Crescent
Winnipeg, Manitoba R3J 3T2
Canada
Tel: 1-204-224-4068

Distributed in Brazil by:
Ernesto Reichmann Distribuidora de Livros, Ltda
Rua Coronel Marques 335, Tatuape 03440-000
Sao Paulo,
Brazil

Composition by Wearset, Boldon, Tyne and Wear.
Printed and bound in Great Britain by Biddles Ltd, Guildford and King's Lynn.

Contents

Contributors

Lawrence J Beilin MD FRCP FRACP
Professor of Medicine, University of Western Australia, Department of Medicine, Royal Perth Hospital, Perth, Australia.

Henry R Black MD PhD
Professor of Preventive Medicine, Roberts Professor of Internal Medicine, and Chairman, Department of Preventive Medicine, Rush-Presbyterian-St Luke's Medical Center, Rush University, Chicago IL, USA.

Hans R Brunner MD
Professor, Division of Hypertension and Vascular Medicine, Center Hospitalier Universitaire, Vaudois, Lausanne, Switzerland.

Michel Burnier MD
Professor, Division of Hypertension and Vascular Medicine, Center Hospitalier Universitaire, Vaudois, Lausanne, Switzerland.

William J Elliott MD PhD
Professor of Preventive Medicine, Internal Medicine, and Pharmacology, Department of Preventive Medicine, Rush Medical College of Rush University, at Rush-Presbyterian-St Luke's Medical Center, Chicago IL, USA.

Ehud Grossman MD
Internal Medicine D, The Chaim Sheba Medical Center, Tel Hashomer, Israel.

Rodney Jackson MD
Professor of Epidemiology and Head, Department of Community Health, Faculty of Medicine and Health Science, The University of Auckland, Auckland, New Zealand.

Franz H Messerli MD
Department of Internal Medicine, Section on Hypertensive Diseases, Ochsner Clinic and Alton Ochsner Medical Foundation, New Orleans LA, USA.

Jan A Staessen MD
Study Coordinating Center, Hypertension and Cardiovascular Rehabilitation Unit, Department of Molecular and Cardiovascular Research, University of Leuven, Leuven, Belgium.

Preface

As might be expected for the most common condition seen in clinical practice among non-pregnant adults, hypertension is under intense study, both in basic and applied research. Advances, fundamental and often immediately applicable to clinical practice, are forthcoming at a steadily increasing pace. Therefore, the need for a frequent up-to-date review of these advances is obvious. *Hypertension Therapy Annual*, hopefully the first to be published on a yearly basis, is designed to meet that need.

When asked to serve as editor, I chose those topics of greatest importance wherein significant advances had recently been made. I then chose authors who were directly involved in the studies which gave rise to these advances. Their contributions in the following seven chapters add up to a book which should be of immense value to all who read it, in turn helping practitioners in providing more effective treatment of their many patients with hypertension.

Norman M Kaplan MD
Dallas TX
January 2000

1

The current inadequate control of hypertension: how can we do better?

William J Elliott

Introduction

Hypertension is an easily diagnosed and eminently modifiable risk factor for adverse cardiovascular and renal outcomes, including death, stroke, myocardial infarction, and dialysis or renal transplantation.[1] Despite the discovery of a simple, non-invasive, and accurate method of measuring blood pressure more than 100 years ago and abundant evidence that reducing blood pressure effectively prevents many adverse health outcomes, there is recent evidence that elevated blood pressure is being managed suboptimally.[1]

Suboptimal hypertension control in the USA

The USA is privileged to have a government that allocates some of its resources to ongoing assessments of the health of its population. One of the largest efforts of this kind is the National Health and Nutritional Evaluation Survey (NHANES), which has periodically surveyed a large cross-section of the population to learn of their attitudes and performance regarding several health-related behaviors. Some of the results from these surveys, as well as data from the American Heart Association, are shown in *Fig. 1.1*. In 1972, when the National High Blood Pressure Education Program was inaugurated, there were approximately 40 million hypertensives in the USA, of whom only about 6.5 million (16%) were controlled. At that time, there were only 21 medications available for the treatment of hypertension, some of which were associated with side effects that troubled people more than the condition itself did. During the past 25 years, there has been a quadrupling of the number of drugs that are useful in lowering blood pressure, but unfortunately, a proportional increase in the percentage of hypertensive patients whose blood pressure is controlled has not been seen.

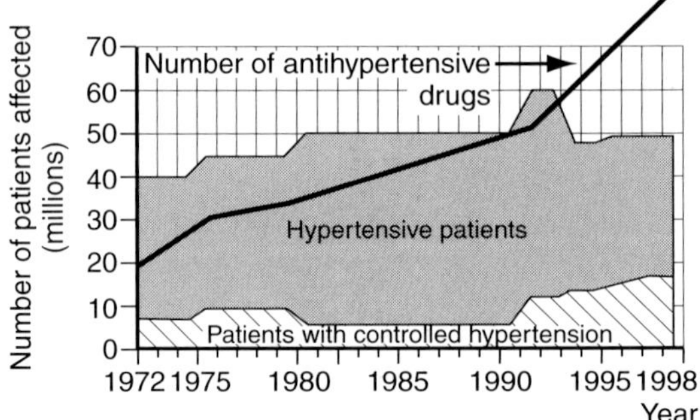

Figure 1.1

Temporal trends in the number of available antihypertensive agents, the prevalence of hypertension, and control of hypertension in the USA, based on NHANES data and American Heart Association estimates.[3]

The most recent data from NHANES III, Part 2, collected from 1991 to 1994, indicate that only 27.4% of hypertensive patients in the USA have controlled blood pressure, even using the 'old' (and now outdated) criteria of <140 mmHg for systolic blood pressure and <90 mmHg for diastolic blood pressure.[1] Although the percentage of hypertensives with controlled blood pressure is higher now than it was in surveys using the same methodology done in the late 1970s and early 1980s, it is currently lower than even the 29% found in 1989–1991.[2] Current estimates are that over 35 million people in the USA are at risk of otherwise preventable cardiovascular events owing to their uncontrolled, elevated blood pressure.

As is typical of large governmental-sponsored surveys, data from NHANES III, Part 2 can be viewed in a number of different ways. On the 'positive side', the percentage of hypertensives who are aware of their elevated blood pressure has continued to increase in the USA since 1972. Similarly, the percentage who are taking steps (including medication) to control their hypertension has also improved, especially in comparison to the first NHANES survey. The improvement in both of these parameters has been cited as being proof that 'the war on hypertension' is being won. Sadly, however, the most important parameter that is likely to have an impact on the public health is neither the number who are aware of their hypertension nor the number taking steps to improve it, but rather the percentage whose blood pressure is under control.

There are several different explanations proposed for the apparent 'fall-off' in the prevalence of controlled hypertension. Many have negatively cited the duration of the public education campaign against hypertension ('the silent killer'), which has now formally exceeded 25 years. Most people in the USA dislike wars in general, but long wars are particularly abhorrent. The recent Gulf War lasted approximately 3 days, but was still too long, in the view of the US electorate. The 'war on hypertension' declared by the NHBPEP in 1972 is therefore seen as being unsustainable, with an inevitable loss of interest even among those affected and their physicians. The attention span of most people in the USA is said to be relatively short, even if the discussion is pertinent to a health risk that directly affects them. A second explanation for the drop-off in controlled hypertension in the USA presupposes that 'the business of America is business', and attempts to relate all national behaviors to commerce. Careful observers of the national economy point out that major strides are made in many public health arenas if there are profits to be made, when more advertisements and more attention is focused on a given area. Current estimates are that approximately $US8.2 billion is spent in the USA on antihypertensive medications, which is 26% of the total cost of treating hypertension.[3] Since the majority of antihypertensive medications are no longer protected by patents and are susceptible to generic substitution, less emphasis is being given to the development of new antihypertensive drugs by the pharmaceutical industry. Their managing directors believe the market is already 'flooded' with 85 approved agents, and the development of any new drug is expected to cost $US350 million just to receive approval from the Food and Drug Administration for marketing. Because the profit-making motive has been largely removed from antihypertensive drug development, many companies that were formerly heavily involved in the process have shifted their focus. Many have found solace (and high profits) in developing cholesterol-lowering medications, the rationale for which is quite similar to what was found in the antihypertensive therapeutic arena about 15–20 years ago.

Correlation of poor blood pressure control and adverse US vital statistics data

One of the great victories in public health in the USA has been the impressive reduction in age-adjusted mortality from cardiovascular causes since 1972. Current estimates (based on vital statistics data reported to the National Center for Health Statistics, Center for Disease Control and Prevention, adjusted for the American population distribution in 1940) indicate that, from 1972 to 1996, there has been a 59% reduction in stroke mortality and a 53% reduction in coronary heart disease mortality.[1] Although some of this trend clearly began before 1972 and although some of the improvement can certainly be attributed to better eating habits, less cigarette smoking, and lowered blood cholesterol values, many authorities point to strides made in hypertension management as being at least partly responsible for this improvement in mortality rates.[4]

Although this encouraging trend is obvious when one looks at the long-term results, much more disturbing details come to light when one focuses only on recent data. The sex-specific mortality rates for cardio-vascular disease for 1988–1995 are shown in *Fig. 1.2*, with the most

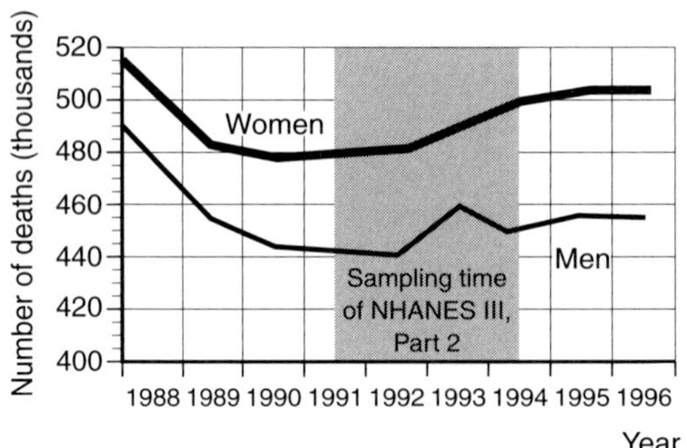

Figure 1.2

Number of deaths from cardiovascular disease, 1988–1996, for women and men. The shaded area corresponds to the sampling time of NHANES III, Part 2. Data adapted from the American Heart Association.[3]

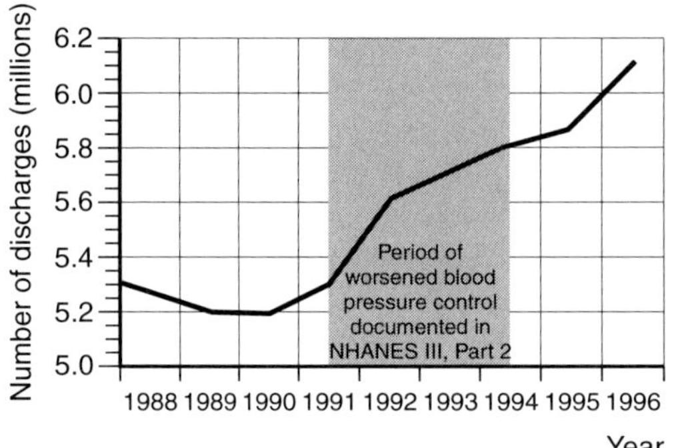

Figure 1.3

Number of hospital discharges for cardiovascular diseases in the USA, 1988–1996. The shaded area corresponds to the period of worsened blood pressure control documented in NHANES III, Part 2. Data adapted from the American Heart Association.[3]

recent years being of specific concern. Despite the continuous and gradual decline in age-adjusted cardiovascular mortality from 1972 onward, 1992 was the first year in 20 years for which there was an *increase* in cardiovascular mortality for both men and women; this trend has continued nearly unabated for each year from 1993 to 1996. It has been suggested that the lack of blood pressure control seen in NHANES III, Part 2 (surveyed during 1991–1994) has contributed to the increase in cardiovascular morbidity and mortality demonstrated in national vital statistics at about the same time.

However, health-care economists have few concerns about mortality, however, since dead people have no further need for health-care resources. Substantially more frightening to those who monitor Medicare expenditures and health maintenance organization profits are the recent data regarding cardiovascular hospitalizations (*Fig. 1.3*), which accounted for $US124 million (70%) of the $US178 million in direct costs for cardiovascular disease in 1999.[3] The recent trends for hospitalizations for coronary heart disease and stroke, and the incidence of end-stage renal disease are very similar: there is a clear increase in these

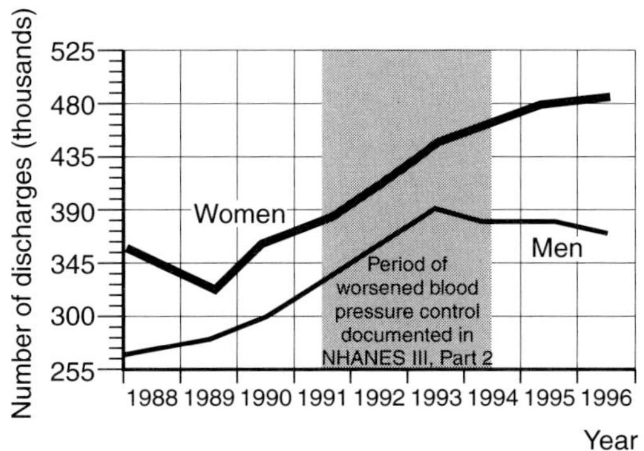

Figure 1.4

Number of discharges from hospitals for congestive heart failure, USA, 1988–1996, for women and men. The shaded area corresponds to the period of worsened blood pressure control documented in NHANES III, Part 2. Data adapted from the American Heart Association.[3]

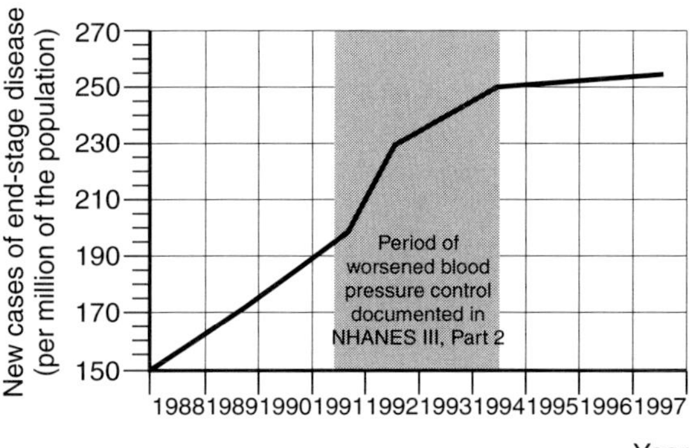

Figure 1.5

Incidence of end-stage renal disease (dialysis or renal transplant) in the USA, 1988–1997. The shaded area corresponds to the time of worsened blood pressure control documented in NHANES III, Part 2. Data adapted from the US Renal Data System.[6]

expensive outcomes at about the time that hypertension control in the USA deteriorated (as documented in the NHANES III, Part 2 results).

The most troubling feature (in terms of total national expenditures) is the annual number of hospitalizations for heart failure (*Fig. 1.4*). Since 1980, heart failure has become the most common reason for hospitalization in the USA among patients over 65 years of age. Despite great advances in treatment strategies, there continue to be increasing numbers of both men and women whose quantity and quality of life are severely reduced by heart failure. A recent meta-analysis has suggested that controlling blood pressure is probably the single most effective preventive therapy for heart failure, with an efficacy rate exceeding 90%.[5] The annual incidence of end-stage renal disease (*Fig. 1.5*) shows a similar concomitant increase in slope during the 1991–1994 time period when blood pressure was not well controlled across the USA.[6]

To summarize recent trends in the USA: there has been a substantive drop-off in the control of hypertension in the general population, which may be one reason why vital statistics show a temporally related increase in cardiovascular morbidity and mortality.

Suboptimal hypertension control in other countries

World-wide, the results of surveys of blood pressure control in populations show an even more dismal picture. An entire conference held in Ottawa, Canada in mid-1995 estimated that less than 15% of the world's hypertensives have achieved control of their blood pressure, even using simple (and, in today's world, probably suboptimal) definitions of 'control'. Geographically, the closest country to the USA that surveys its population regarding the prevalence of controlled hypertension is Canada, which uses a survey methodology very similar to the NHANES in the USA. Both essentially target randomly selected adults from census data, with blood pressures measured by trained nurses doing home visits. The results of the recent Canadian Home Health Survey of 23,129 randomly selected Canadian adults showed controlled hypertension (<140 mmHg systolic and <90 mmHg diastolic) in only 22% of the participants.[7] These data suggest that despite the putative advantages of the Canadian National Healthcare System (which is highly regarded by people in the USA who favor a 'single-payer' system for US citizens),[8] blood pressure control rates are even lower north of the Canadian–US border than they are south of it.

Two other major surveys of European patients are not easy to compare to these North American data. The recent Cardiomonitor survey was performed by performing chart audits of physicians' offices in Spain, France, the UK, and Germany. These countries are remarkable because of their highly evolved systems of health-care delivery, in which the government shoulders a major part of the financing. Among the 23,339 charts reviewed, 37% of patients were found to have their blood pressure under control.[9] This percentage is not directly comparable to the North American surveys because of differences in where blood pressures were measured and who measured them, and in what constitutes controlled hypertension. (Europeans typically favor the previous World Health Organization (WHO)–International Society of Hypertension (ISH) definition of 160/90 mmHg, which is considerably less stringent than recommendations from the US Joint National Committee.[10]) Another population-based survey of hypertension control was done near Gubbio, Italy, where patients pay more of the cost of care than in the countries selected for the Cardiomonitor survey. In this review of 3,238 patients' charts, controlled blood pressure (less than 160/90 mmHg) was found only in 18% of patients.[11]

Suggestions from the sixth report of the US Joint National Committee

The sixth report of the US Joint National Committee on Prevention, Detection, Evaluation, and Treatment of High Blood Pressure (JNC VI) contains some new recommendations regarding blood pressure control in individual patients, as well as a review of much of the foregoing information about the deterioration of hypertension control in the USA.[1] JNC VI provides, for the first time, a classification scheme for blood pressure that includes the term 'optimal' blood pressure, which is intended for people who achieve a blood pressure below 120/70 mmHg (i.e. 120 mmHg systolic *and* 70 mmHg diastolic) without the benefit of antihypertensive drug therapy. It is meant to reassure those who have enviably low blood pressures that they need not be concerned about untoward risk of having 'too low' a blood pressure, but instead should take steps to keep the blood pressure at this desirable level. Secondly, the classification scheme of JNC VI continues (as did its predecessor) the equal weight of systolic and diastolic blood pressure. For nearly 20 years, blood pressure in the USA was classified solely by the diastolic reading; now large databases from insurance companies, and data from clinical trials[12–14] have proven the importance of controlling not only the diastolic blood pressure, but the systolic blood pressure as well.[15]

The second major change in JNC VI (compared to its predecessor) is that it recommends 'risk stratification' before the initiation of antihypertensive drug therapy (*Table 1.1*). This new scheme holds out two major hopes for control of hypertension, both of which are expected to improve the cost-effectiveness of treatment.

First, for very low-risk patients (e.g. the young female with only an elevated blood pressure and no other cardiovascular risk factors), it is recommended that potentially expensive antihypertensive drug therapy should be withheld for 1 year, during which time lifestyle modifications should be the only treatment. This is considered both ethical and cost-effective because the absolute risk of adverse cardiovascular disease events in young, healthy, and otherwise low-risk hypertensives is extremely small in the short term; it is likely to improve cost-effectiveness because no drug therapy will be prescribed for these patients (or 'wasted', in the eyes of many payers) since they are very unlikely to have a stroke or cardiovascular event during the next year anyway.[16]

The 'flip side' of this recommendation is that high-risk hypertensives ('risk group C': those with two or more traditional cardiovascular risk factors or with diabetes mellitus) should be immediately started on antihypertensive drug therapy, even if their blood pressure is in the 'high normal' range (130–139/85–89 mmHg). The governing hypothesis here is that initiating therapy in high-risk hypertensives at a lower threshold will put the medications to excellent use in a population that is very likely to benefit from them; this also should improve cost-effectiveness of treatment in the long term.[17]

The impact of 'white-coat' hypertension

The discussion of 'white-coat' hypertension in JNC VI may be of lesser importance to the general population, but it may have major consequences

Table 1.1 Risk stratification before treatment of blood pressure[1]

Blood pressure stage		Risk group		
		A	B	C
	Number of risk factors	0	1 (no diabetes mellitus)	≥2 (or diabetes mellitus)
	Target organ damage	Absent	Absent	Present
	Cardiovascular disease	Absent	Absent	Present
High normal		Lifestyle modification forever	Lifestyle modification forever	Drug therapy
Stage 1		Lifestyle modification for 12 months	Lifestyle modification for 6 months	Drug therapy
Stage 2		Drug therapy	Drug therapy	Drug therapy
Stage 3		Drug therapy	Drug therapy	Drug therapy

for blood pressure control rates. Research during the past 10–15 years has indicated that approximately 20–25% of people have a higher blood pressure when it is measured in a health-care setting (e.g. a hospital, an emergency department, or a physician's office) than when it is measured while they are performing their usual daily activities. There are now normative data from more than 5000 normal people; these data provide an upper limit for average daily blood pressure (obtained by ambulatory blood pressure monitoring (ABPM)).[18] Even more important are data that suggest that patients whose blood pressure is elevated only in the physician's office have *lower* rates of cardiovascular morbidity and mortality than patients whose blood pressure is elevated both at home and in the office setting.[19] These studies suggest that data about hypertension control derived from chart reviews may overestimate the proportion of uncontrolled hypertension because of the 'white-coat' phenomenon; the counterargument is that surveys of blood pressure control in physicians' offices obviously do not include patients who are non-compliant with visiting the physician (and these patients are also more likely to be non-compliant in taking their antihypertensive medication, and therefore have elevated blood pressures). JNC VI has at least recognized the phenomenon of 'white-coat' hypertension, although it has not espoused ABPM as a means of evaluating whether or not a given person's elevated blood pressure is due to this phenomenon. Several cost-effectiveness analyses have indicated that, in carefully selected people, ABPM can be done annually and still save money because those patients who are identified as having the 'white-coat' effect will be able to avoid more intensive treatment and its attendant costs.[20]

Still-lower blood pressure goals for treated high-risk patients?

Probably the most important recommendation by JNC VI, from the perspective of achieving control of blood pressure in populations, is the new target blood pressure levels for specific, high-risk populations. For most of the (otherwise low-risk) hypertensive population, the recommended blood pressure target is <140/90 mmHg. This is quite congruent with the findings of the Hypertension Optimal Treatment (HOT) Study,[21] which provided 136.2/84.6 mmHg as the 'optimal' treated blood pressure level for long-term avoidance of cardiovascular events. For higher-risk hypertensives with either diabetes mellitus or established renal impairment, the blood pressure goal of <130/85 mmHg is recommended. Finally, for patients with >1 g of proteinuria, a still lower blood pressure goal of <125/75 mmHg should be attained.

There are two more recent studies that have corroborated the recommendation of JNC VI for diabetic patients. In the HOT study, 1501 diabetics were enrolled and the best results (in avoiding cardiovascular events) were found in the group randomized to the lowest blood pressure goal

($\leq$80 mmHg diastolic blood pressure; p <0.005 for the trend across the three blood pressure targets).[21] Similarly, in the United Kingdom Prospective Diabetes Study 38, the group randomized to the lower blood pressure goal (target of 150/85 mmHg) had 32% fewer deaths, 44% fewer strokes, 24% fewer diabetes-related end-points, and 37% fewer microvascular end-points than the control group (whose target blood pressure was initially 180/105 mmHg).[22]

The impact of these changes in JNC VI on blood pressure control rates is, unfortunately, likely to be *negative*, in that high-risk patients who were formerly considered to have controlled hypertension (blood pressure <140/90 mmHg) will now need lower blood pressure to be considered 'controlled'. There are already some data from locales and managed care organizations in the USA that have identified a much lower rate of controlled hypertension in diabetic or renally impaired hypertensives than in the broader population of hypertensives in the same medical care system.[23] Despite this concern, the impact of these recommendations from JNC VI are likely to improve the cost-effectiveness of the treatment of hypertension, because it will withhold expensive treatment from those who are unlikely to benefit (at least in the short term) and recommends more intensive treatment of those at high risk of very expensive strokes or myocardial infarctions.

Improving blood pressure control by changing public perceptions

Most public health authorities would recognize the National High Blood Pressure Education Program (NHBPEB) as the most effective campaign in changing public perception of a major chronic health problem in the USA over the past 25 years. Their approach was essentially copied by the National Cholesterol Education Program about 15 years after the NHBPEP program began. Since 1972, there has been a large drop in age-adjusted mortality both from stroke (a decrease of 62%) and from coronary artery disease (a decrease of 55%), which many have attributed to the greater awareness of hypertension.[1] Many believe that it is now time to refocus our efforts on hypertension, both because we have so many relatively inexpensive, easily tolerated antihypertensive agents available and because the recent vital statistics data discussed above suggest that attention to controlling this very important cardiovascular risk factor has waned.

The greatest difficulty is focusing the public's attention on this issue. Hypertension is seen by many people as being an 'old' (i.e., outdated, passé, boring) issue. There are, however, several aspects of hypertension and its therapy that can be repackaged and that may well restore the public's interest in this area.

One recent study that is likely to be widely quoted for some time and to help people understand the virtues of controlled hypertension is the Hypertension Optimal Treatment (HOT) Study.[21] Many people have the unfortunate opinion that they are protecting themselves from cardiovascular risk if they take antihypertensive drug therapy, irrespective of the blood pressure reduction achieved. While it is likely that taking nearly any antihypertensive drug will be better than taking no medication (as seen in two recent studies that used placebo as the control group, probably the last time this can be done in patients whose blood pressure is >160/90 mmHg[13,14]), there are now data that suggest that, especially in high-risk patients, a lower blood pressure leads to a longer and more productive life. This was most clearly shown for the diabetics in HOT and UKPDS (see pages 51–52), but it has also been seen in the Modification of Diet in Renal Disease (MDRD) study of patients with established renal impairment.[24] In the general population, however, there has been reluctance on the part of both physicians and patients to achieve recommended blood pressure goals, with one popular extreme viewpoint suggesting that too vigorous a lowering of blood pressure is associated with greater risk in the long-term.[25,26] This 'J-shaped curve' hypothesis was directly tested in the HOT study by randomizing 18,790 hypertensive patients from 26 countries to one of three diastolic blood pressure goals ($\leq$90 mmHg, $\leq$85 mmHg, or $\leq$80 mmHg), treating them with relatively well-tolerated antihypertensive agents, and following them for 3.8 years (on average). The most interesting aspect of the study design was not widely reported initially and may still be underappreciated by the general physician and hypertensive population. The duration of the study was actually increased by nearly 2 years during follow-up because the major cardiovascular event rates (stroke, myocardial infarction, or cardiovascular death) were about 40% lower than anticipated. The expected rates of these adverse events were based on estimates from previous studies of older antihypertensive agents (primarily diuretics, but some β-blockers);[27] the very subtle conclusion from the overall study was that the medications used to control blood pressure in this study were more effective than originally planned in reducing the risk of cardiovascular events. Sadly, this 'message' was not very effectively conveyed during the initial 'media blitz' associated with the announcement of the final results of the HOT study.

The more accurately reported 'message' from the HOT study was that the lower target blood pressures were not associated with any further increase in cardiovascular risk, although room for some uncertainty regarding the appropriate target blood pressure for uncomplicated hypertensives still exists. Public perception often changes after an extreme is explored and shown to be beneficial; this principle may well underlie the popularity of the extreme dietary and hygienic measures espoused by Dr Dean Ornish (a well-known US authority on preventive cardiology), only some of which have eventually been adopted by at-risk individuals. One hope is that the HOT study results will convince many hypertensives that 'lower is better' with regard to their blood pressure, and since increasing doses of many of the drugs used for antihypertensive drug treatment do not cause a great increase in the incidence of adverse effects, patients may be willing to intensify their antihypertensive drug therapy and achieve the lower blood pressure goal.

The second arena in which changing public opinion may eventually lead to improved rates of blood pressure control is the public's opinion of some of the newer antihypertensive agents. Concerns about 'alternative therapy' (the terminology used in JNC V for angiotensin converting enzyme (ACE) inhibitors, calcium antagonists, α-blockers, and newer drugs) were expressed in 1993, when these agents were not on the list of 'preferred' treatment for hypertension.[28] Despite the lack of long-term safety data for many of the agents and a near-complete lack of data demonstrating benefits of these drugs in reducing cardiovascular events, physicians and patients in the USA did not follow the JNC V recommendation to 'prefer' diuretics or β-blockers.[29]

The issue of the long-term safety of the most popular drug class for hypertension was brought to the public's attention by a news conference held in San Antonio, Texas, USA at 4.00 p.m. central standard time on 11 March 1995, at which it was announced that calcium antagonists were associated with a 60% increased risk of acute myocardial infarction in a case–control study.[30] This was widely reported by all television and radio networks in the USA within minutes, and it caught the public's attention in a major way. This allegation was followed in a few months by several other reports drawing attention to potential harm associated with taking these medications, including an increased risk of death in patients taking higher doses of nifedipine,[31] an increased risk of bleeding in a small clinical trial of post-thoracotomy patients and in several epidemiological databases,[32] and (perhaps most worryingly) an increased future risk of cancer (and even specifically breast cancer[33]) in cohorts of elderly patients gathered for epidemiological studies of other diseases.[34] Each of these reports received widespread media attention, and they may be one reason why many patients have discontinued their antihypertensive drug treatment (so rendering their blood pressure less well controlled) over the past few years.[35]

Only recently have the results of clinical trials using newer antihypertensive agents been reported; sadly, there still seems to be more attention focused on the smaller, but negative, studies than on the larger, and more positive, studies, which may be more generalizable to the hypertensive population. The two studies that were widely reported to show difficulties with calcium antagonists (as first-line therapy) were the Appropriate Blood pressure Control in Diabetes (ABCD)[36] study, about which ABC News, on 22 February 1998, broke the 'Inglefinger Rule' of the *New England Journal of Medicine*'s embargo on publicity before publication; this brought the study results a great deal of notoriety. This report, based on a 2×2 factorial design study of two levels of blood pressure control and two initial treatments for hypertension (nisoldipine or enalapril) in 470 diabetics from Colorado, USA, suggested a 9.5-fold increased risk of acute myocardial infarction for the group treated initially with nisoldipine. Aside from the small total of affected patients (25 versus 5) over 5 years and the separate analysis of this secondary end-point, there were large differences between groups in use of the 'add-on' medications, which were more commonly given to the enalapril group because it had poorer blood pressure control without metoprolol or hydrochlorothiazide. The second report to suggest harm in treating diabetics with calcium antagonists, the Fosinopril Amlodipine Cardiovascular Events Trial,[37] was an unusual clinical trial in that the 380 Italian patients whose blood pressure was not controlled on the initial treatment were given the second agent in combination with the originally assigned drug. Although in the group initially assigned to amlodipine, 27 patients experienced a cardiovascular event (compared to only 10 patients in the group originally assigned to fosinopril; $p < 0.03$), the best results were seen in the group that received both drugs (four events) and, presumably, had the lowest blood pressures. This report generated much interest among diabetics and endocrinologists, and it caused the Data Safety and Monitoring Boards of two very large studies that provide calcium antagonists to large numbers of diabetic patients to examine their data for similar evidence of harm. These disturbing findings were not replicated in either ALLHAT (42,516 patients) or CONVINCE (8,245 patients at that time); both studies continued their treatment and follow-up without alteration of the originally-designed protocol.

Recently, several studies have demonstrated the efficacy of some of the newer medications in reducing cardiovascular events. The first is the HOT study, which had no control group but did show a better-than-expected reduction in cardiovascular events (see pages 11–12). The second and third studies are very similar: the Systolic Hypertension in Europe trial (Syst-Eur)[13] and the Systolic Hypertension in China trial (Syst-China).[14] Both studied older patients with primarily elevations in systolic blood pressure, giving half of the patients placebo and half of the patients nitrendipine (as initial treatment). The allocation of patients was done differently in the two studies, based on local tradition: in Syst-Eur the patients were randomized, but in Syst-China the allocations were made in sequential fashion (which is the custom in China, where 'leaving things to chance' is considered unlucky, if not unwise). The second-step medication was also different between the two studies: Syst-Eur used enalapril, followed by hydrochlorothiazide; Syst-China used captopril and then (if needed) hydrochlorothiazide. A third differences was the way the studies ended: Syst-Eur was stopped prematurely by the Data Safety and

Monitoring Board because of the large difference in stroke rates between treatment groups, but Syst-China was allowed to continue until its planned conclusion with an average of 5 years of follow-up.

Despite these differences between studies, the main results were nearly identical. Syst-Eur showed a 42% reduction in stroke incidence in the actively treated group; Syst-China's result was a 38% reduction in stroke incidence in the actively treated group. Similar reductions in many of the cardiovascular events that were secondary end-points in these trials were also noted with treatment, and there was no evidence of an increase in death, bleeding, or cancer among the patients treated initially with the calcium antagonist.

A recent subgroup analysis of the Syst-Eur diabetic patients has been published,[40] and (despite some potentially inappropriate comparisons to data from SHEP,[12] which was collected some years before the Syst-Eur study) it calls attention to the greater improvements in prognosis in elderly hypertensive diabetics when they are treated initially with a calcium antagonist compared to when they are initially treated with a diuretic (as in SHEP). The major conclusion of this subgroup analysis, however, was that diabetics did not appear to have a worsened prognosis when their hypertension was treated with the calcium antagonist, which contradicts the much smaller ABCD and FACET studies. By 2002 or 2003, the results of WHO–ISH Collaborative Group should be available. This group is collecting individual patient-based data from 31 studies of newer versus older antihypertensive drugs, which should be able to answer this question definitively.[41]

The earliest of these studies of newer versus older antihypertensive drugs to be finished and report its results was the CAPPPP (CAPtopril Primary Prevention Project), which randomized hypertensive patients to either captopril (50%) or (a physician-directed choice of) a diuretic or a β-blocker (50% together).[42] The results showed a roughly equivalent reduction in cardiovascular events, although more of the patients treated with captopril had strokes (perhaps because of a maldistribution of stroke risk factors before randomization) and more of the patients treated with the more traditional regimen developed diabetes. The main 'message' to many patients through the media was unfortunately not that lowering blood pressure (by whatever means) is effective in reducing cardiovascular risk, but rather that the newer drug was sadly (at least in the unadjusted analyses) associated with a *higher* risk of stroke. The implication of this experience is important for those who are charged with announcing the conclusions of the many comparative studies that are still ongoing: it would be most helpful to present all the conclusions in a way that makes clear that lowering blood pressure is indeed helpful in reducing cardiovascular risk.

A third method of improving the public's perception of antihypertensive drug therapy is to demonstrate benefits with certain antihypertensive agents in concomitant disease states that are of great concern to the populace. The recent suggestions that ACE inhibitors may prevent cancer,[43] that some antihypertensive agents may reduce the risk of Alzheimer's disease,[44] and that β-blockers after a myocardial infarction reduce the risk of death in the population at large[45] are all interpreted by many members of the public to be advantageous and may well improve some people's opinions sufficiently to increase the odds that they will actually consume the medication.

Improving compliance

One of the most disturbing issues related to the control of hypertension is the very large number of patients who are initially given antihypertensive drug therapy but who discontinue it, even after a short period of time. Recent estimates from a database of over 1 million beneficiaries in the UK of a pharmacy benefits plan indicate that over 50% of patients discontinue their antihypertensive drug within 6 months of starting it.[46] This statistic is very disturbing to those who must pay for health care, since the cost-effectiveness of such treatment is infinite: the patients (or their payers) incur all the cost of the treatment, but derive none of its benefits. One of the current disease management plans that is popular among pharmacists and pharmacy benefits managers is intended to maximize the benefit of the dispensed drug. Such programs provide many services that presumably make it easier to continue chronic drug therapy, e.g. telephone reminders to patients who are late in refilling prescriptions, the monitoring of blood pressure in pharmacies, the maintenance of close contacts (typically by facsimile transmission) with treating physicians, and the recommending of less expensive dosage forms of medication, among other measures.

The current estimates of the health-care resources related to hypertension that are wasted as a result of non-compliance with drug therapy are staggering (*Table 1.2*), and amount to about 10% of the money spent on hypertension therapy.[47] These estimates do not include any indirect costs, which are even higher; they include not only the cost of pills that go uningested after being dispensed from the pharmacy but also the cost of medical care and disability or survivorship payments disbursed to those who, as a consequence of not taking their antihypertensive medications as prescribed, sadly die or suffer a stroke or myocardial infarction. These estimates also do not include the excess risk of cardiovascular events following acute withdrawal from certain antihypertensive agents (e.g. β-blockers, clonidine), which occurs when the medications are taken on an intermittently discontinuous basis. The health-care economist would point out that some of these costs to the health-care system of non-compliance would be reduced by the cost of

Table 1.2 Estimates of direct costs of non-compliance for hypertension in the USA

Approximate cost ($US) in 1996	Item
42 million	2–12% of hospitalizations
24 million	23% of nursing home placements
63 million	9% of prescriptions going unfilled
65 million	10% of medical advice unheeded
194 million	Total cost (9% of total direct cost of hypertension in 1996)

medications and visits to health-care providers which are not spent by persons who decide not to take their medications; the balance between the two is currently controversial.

One way of improving the prevalence of controlled hypertension is to bring more resources to bear on the problem of non-compliance with antihypertensive medications. As mentioned above, this has been a major focus of several approaches to the problem of hypertension, and it is a major issue of great importance to pharmacists and managed care pharmacy benefits managers. They have developed a number of ways of improving compliance with medication, some of which have been shown in clinical trials to lead to more predictable taking of medication that is more in accordance with the original prescription. Some of these are summarized in *Table 1.3*.

Similar to the problem of medication compliance is the issue of visit adherence (defined as returning *as scheduled* to a site of health-care delivery for intermittent monitoring). Many have noted that, after a short period of enthusiasm for controlling hypertension, manifested by a few months of fulfilled appointments, there is often a decline in appointment-keeping. Some centers have reported that as few as 2–10% of patients return to the office of their health-care provider 1 year after their original appointment, even though the medical problem (e.g. hypertension) that was the reason for the original visit has not gone away completely. Several suggestions have been made that can help to rectify the large numbers of patients who become 'lost to follow-up'; these include:

(a) establishing an identified health-care provider as the primary care-giver;
(b) designating specific appointment times reserved for the individual patient;

Table 1.3 Methods of improving compliance

Educate the patient about the reason for the medications and their proper use
Improve patient's social support network (e.g. spouse or caregiver)
Increase patient's autonomy and involvement in decision-making (when appropriate), including home blood pressure monitoring
Remove barriers to compliance with pill-taking (e.g. by avoiding large or bad-tasting pills)
Simplify the therapeutic regimen (minimize the number of pills, frequency of pill-taking, and the inconvenience of pill-taking)
Integrate pill-taking into activities of daily living (e.g. brushing teeth)
Provide a positive attitude and positive reinforcement about achieving therapeutic goals

(c) using well-tolerated therapy that is tailored to the individual patient being treated;

(d) using relatively inexpensive therapies, the cost of which is reimbursed by other parties (whenever possible);

(e) reminding the patient by telephone or letter of forthcoming appointments; and

(f) having health-care information available from the health-care provider by telephone, fax, or electronic mail outside regular office hours.

Several of these interventions have been shown to improve appointment-keeping behavior in clinical studies.

There remains a great deal of work to be done to provide optimal delivery of both medications and health care according to the prescribed schedule. The 'systems approaches' to these problems provide the highest probability of improvement, but they may require a substantial investment in technology before their implementation can be widespread. Much current research is focused on this area, and results are expected in a few years.

Quality indicators may improve rates of blood pressure control

One of the major forces in health care today is the quest for quality (and its improvement).[48] This issue has become a driving force in managed care systems, primarily because it affects enrollment, retention, and profits of large healthcare organizations.[49] Although there is a great deal of discussion about which group (e.g. the National Committee for Quality Assurance, the Health Care Financing Authority) will provide the 'yardsticks' by which quality of health-care delivery will be measured, there is little doubt that such assessments have a large impact on the therapeutic areas that are targeted for scrutiny.[48] Although hypertension control rates are currently being assessed only in large health-care delivery systems as 'test cases', this will soon change. After the year 2000, when the Healthplan Employer Data Information Set 3.5 guidelines are implemented,[50] we can expect a much greater emphasis on hypertension control rates, since this will be one of the 'quality indicators' reported by large health-care organizations. Currently, Healthy People 2000 (a cooperative effort of legislators, governmental policymakers, private citizens, and regulators) has set the goal for the USA to achieve control of hypertension in 50% of the affected people surveyed.[51] Most reports (including NHANES III, Part 2) currently find a far lower prevalence of controlled hypertension than this. One of the benefits of placing hypertension control rates on the menu of parameters surveyed as an indicator of health-care quality is that we will soon have much more data from many organized health-care systems about their ability to control hypertension.[48] The other major benefit is that, since these 'quality indicators' are often used by both end-users and purchasers of health care as a reason for enrolling in plans that provide 'quality care', there will soon be much more attention focused on individual physicians, health-care service organizations, and health maintenance organizations to improve their rates of hypertension control.[48]

There are many ways in which physicians and managed care organizations can be influenced to improve hypertension control rates, one of which is directly linked to reimbursement.[52] There are several current proposals that would reward health maintenance organizations for achieving 'quality benchmarks' by either paying higher premiums or guaranteeing greater enrollment. Thus, there is a great incentive for organized health systems to begin to focus attention on controlling hypertension.

The incentives are even greater at the level of the individual physician. Several plans 'reward' the physician for achieving 'quality benchmarks' (typically assessed by chart review). Even more likely to capture the attention of physicians is the prospect of a reduction in income or even dismissal from a given health plan because of failure to achieve a recommended level of 'quality care'. One widely practiced incentive for individual physicians bases the provision of a 'holdback' (some fraction of monies that are routinely withheld from payments for services rendered), which can be released to the physician if the year's review of quality indicators passes established thresholds. In some locales, hypertension control rates are a part of the equation used to decide whether the physician recoups the 'holdback' at the end of the year; typically the 'payline' is set at levels higher than the Healthy People 2000 goal. Although there are potential problems with physicians (and other health-care providers) recording blood pressure readings that may be biased toward lower numbers (which would obviously make it more likely that the 'holdback' would be provided), there is little doubt that both patients and their physicians are likely to become much more aware of their blood pressures after this system is implemented.

Adopting better-tolerated antihypertensive drug therapy

One of the theories why so few patients remain on their originally prescribed antihypertensive drug therapies holds that many of the traditionally recommended drug classes cause frequent symptomatic side effects, which are often less well-tolerated than the symptomless elevation in blood pressure. Some believe that diuretics or β-blockers are more likely than calcium antagonists, ACE inhibitors, or α-blockers to cause adverse effects that will be recognized by patients but not often brought to the attention of their physicians. Recent data from randomized clinical trials,[53,54] and large pharmacy databases do not corroborate this conclusion. Nonetheless, one of the reasons why few physicians and patients seem to be following the recommendations of the JNC about the choice of initial antihypertensive drug therapy may be concern about the adverse effects associated with these drug classes.

One of the great hopes for the newest class of oral antihypertensive agents, the angiotensin II receptor blockers, is that these drugs may be very helpful in obtaining better control of hypertension in broad populations than their predecessors. These drugs are typically very well tolerated and do not cause the cough that is seen in 10–15% of people who take an ACE inhibitor.[55] There are some data that suggest that a higher proportion of patients given these drugs persist in their therapy than patients given other classes of antihypertensive medications.[56] Unfortunately, the angiotensin II receptor blockers are all currently priced at levels that are considerably higher than ACE inhibitors (especially generic captopril), and there are therefore large economic incentives to restrict their use to patients who cannot tolerate an ACE inhibitor. There is also the concern that these drugs have not (as yet!) been shown to have the same beneficial effects as the ACE inhibitors, not just in hypertension, but also in heart failure, renal impairment, proteinuria, and diabetes.

Summary

In short, the prevalence of controlled hypertension in many large populations has not yet achieved the goals set by governmental and other authorities. This may be one of the reasons why US vital statistics data have recently shown worsened rates of cardiovascular death, stroke, coronary artery disease, congestive heart failure, and end-stage renal failure, and it bodes ill for the future. Steps that may improve hypertension control include:

(a) making a proper diagnosis of hypertension (with multiple readings at several visits);

(b) improving public awareness and perceptions about the benefits of having lower blood pressure;

(c) demonstrating (to physicians, patients, and payers) the benefits of lower blood pressure in large outcome-based clinical trials;

(d) maximizing compliance with medications and visits to health-care providers;

(e) providing tangible incentives for physicians (and health plans) to control blood pressure; and

(f) using better-tolerated antihypertensive drug therapy.

References

1. The sixth report of the Joint National Committee on Prevention, Detection, Evaluation, and Treatment of High Blood Pressure (JNC VI). Arch Intern Med 1997; 157: 2413–2446.

2. Burt VL, Whelton PK, Roccella EJ *et al*. Prevalence of hypertension in the US adult population: results from the Third National Health and Nutritional Examination survey, 1988–91. Hypertension 1995; 25: 305–313.

3. American Heart Association. 1999 Heart and Stroke Facts, Statistical Update. Dallas, Texas, USA: American Heart Association, 1999.

4. Mosterd A, D'Agostino RB, Silbershatz H *et al*. Trends in the prevalence of hypertension, antihypertensive therapy, and left ventricular hypertrophy from 1950 to 1989. N Engl J Med 1999; 340: 1221–1227.

5. Moser M, Hebert PR. Prevention of disease progression, left ventricular hypertrophy and congestive heart failure in hypertension treatment trials. J Am Coll Cardiol 1996; 27: 1214–1218.

6. US Renal Data System. USRDS 1998 Annual Report. Bethesda, Maryland, USA: US Department of Health and Human Services, National Institute of Diabetes and Digestive and Kidney Disease, 1998.

7. Joffres MR, Ghadirian P, Fodor JG *et al*. Awareness, treatment, and control of hypertension in Canada. Am J Hypertension 1997; 10: 1097–1102.

8. Light DW. Good managed care needs universal health insurance. Ann Intern Med 1999; 130: 686–689.

9. Hosie J, Wiklund I. Managing hypertension in general practice: can we do better? J Human Hypertension 1995; 9 (suppl 2): S15–S18.

10. Fahey TP, Peters TJ. What constitutes controlled hypertension? Patient-based comparison of hypertension guidelines. BMJ 1996; 313: 93–96.

11. Zanchetti A. Antihypertensive therapy: pride and prejudice. J Hypertens 1995; 13: 1522–1528.

12. The SHEP Cooperative Study Group. Prevention of stroke by antihypertensive drug treatment in older persons with isolated systolic hypertension. JAMA 1991; 265: 3255–3264.

13. Staessen JA, Fagard R, Thijs L *et al*. Randomised double-blind

comparison of placebo and active treatment for older patients with isolated systolic hypertension. The Systolic Hypertension in Europe (Syst-Eur) Trial Investigators. Lancet 1997; 350: 757–764.

14. Liu L, Wang J, Gong L *et al.* for the Systolic Hypertension in China (Syst-China) Collaborative Group. Comparison of active treatment and placebo in older Chinese patients with isolated systolic hypertension. J Hypertens 1998; 16: 1823–1829.

15. Elliott WJ. Which blood pressure is more important in the elderly (editorial)? Arch Intern Med 1999; 159: 1165–1166.

16. Elliott WJ. The costs of treating hypertension. In: Epstein M, ed. Calcium Antagonists in Clinical Medicine 2nd edn. Philadelphia, Pennsylvania, USA: Hanley and Belfus, 1998, 513–526.

17. Jönsson BG. Cost-benefit of treating hypertension. J Hypertens Suppl 1994; 12: S65–S75.

18. Staessen JA, O'Brien ET, Atkins N, Amery AM. Short report: ambulatory blood pressure in normotensive compared with hypertensive subjects. The Ad-Hoc Working Group. J Hypertens 1993; 11: 1289–1297.

19. Verdecchia P, Porcellati C, Schillaci G *et al.* Ambulatory blood pressure: an independent predictor of prognosis in essential hypertension. Hypertension 1994; 24: 793–801.

20. Yarows SA, Khoury S, Sowers JR. Cost effectiveness of 24-hour ambulatory blood pressure monitoring in evaluation and treatment of essential hypertension. Am J Hypertens 1994; 7: 464–468.

21. Hansson L, Zanchetti A, Julius S *et al.* on behalf of the HOT Study Group. Effects of intensive blood pressure lowering and low-dose aspirin in patients with hypertension: principal results of the Hypertension Optimal Treatment (HOT) randomised trial. Lancet 1998; 351: 1755–1762.

22. Turner R, Holman R, Stratton I *et al.* for the United Kingdom Prospective Diabetes Study Group. Tight blood pressure control and risk of macrovascular and microvascular complications in type 2 diabetes: UKPDS 38. BMJ 1998; 317: 707–713.

23. Elliott WJ, Toth SJ, Stemer A, Cadwalader J for the Inland/United Steelworkers of America Health Care Network. Detection, treatment, and control of adult hypertension in northwest Indiana. Am J Hypertens 1999; 14: 830–834.

24. Lazarus JM, Bourgoignie JJ, Buckalew VM *et al.* for the Modification of Diet in Renal Disease Study Group. Achievement and safety of a low blood pressure goal in chronic renal disease: the Modification of Diet in Renal Disease Study Group. Hypertension 1997; 29: 641–650.

25. Farnett L, Mulrow CD, Linn WD *et al.* The J-curve phenomenon and the treatment of hypertension. Is there a point beyond which pressure reduction is dangerous? JAMA 1991; 265: 489–495.

26. Fletcher AE, Bulpitt CJ. How far should blood pressure be lowered? N Engl J Med 1992; 326: 251–254.

27. Collins R, Peto R, MacMahon S *et al.* Blood pressure, stroke, and coronary heart disease. Part 2: short-term reductions in blood pressure: overview of randomised drug trials in their epidemiological context. Lancet 1990; 335: 827–838.

28. Weber MA, Laragh JH. Hypertension: steps forward and steps backward. Arch Intern Med 1993; 153: 149–152.

29. Siegel D, Lopez J. Trends in anti-hypertensive drug use in the United States: do the JNC V recommendations affect prescribing? JAMA 1997; 278: 1745–1748.

30. Psaty BM, Heckbert SR, Koepsell TD *et al.* The risk of myocardial infarction associated with antihypertensive drug therapies. JAMA 1995; 274: 620–625.

31. Furberg CD, Psaty BM, Meyer JV. Nifedipine: dose-related increase in mortality in patients with coronary heart disease. Circulation 1995; 92: 1326–1331.

32. Pahor M, Guralnik JM, Furberg CD *et al.* Risk of gastrointestinal haemorrhage with calcium antagonists in hypertensive persons over 67 years old. Lancet 1996; 347: 1061–1065.

33. Fitzpatrick AL, Daling JR, Furberg CD *et al.* Use of calcium channel blockers and breast cancer risk in postmenopausal women. Cancer 1997; 80: 1438–1447.

34. Pahor M, Guralnik JM, Ferrucci L *et al.* Calcium channel blockade and incidence of cancer in aged populations. Lancet 1996; 348: 493–498.

35. Maclure M, Dormuth C, Naumann T *et al.* Influences of educational interventions and adverse news about calcium-channel blockers on first-line prescribing of antihypertensive drugs to elderly people in British Columbia. Lancet 1998; 352: 942–948.

36. Estacio RO, Jeffers BW, Hiatt WR *et al.* The effect of nisoldipine as compared with enalapril on cardiovascular outcomes in patients with non-insulin dependent diabetes and hypertension. N Engl J Med 1998; 335: 645–652.

37. Tatti P, Pahor M, Byington R *et al.* Outcome results of the Fosinopril versus Amlodipine Cardiovascular Events randomized Trial (FACET) in patients with hypertension and NIDDM. Diabetes Care 1998; 21: 597–603.

38. Davis BR, Cutler JA, Gordon DJ *et al.* Rationale and design for the Antihypertensive and Lipid Lowering treatment to prevent Heart Attack Trial (ALLHAT). Am J Hypertens 1996; 9: 342–360.

39. Black HR, Elliott WJ, Neaton JC *et al.* for the CONVINCE Research Group. Rationale and design for the Controlled ONset Verapamil INvestigation of Cardiovascular Endpoints (CONVINCE) trial. Contr Clin Trials 1998; 19: 370–390.

40. Toumilehto J, Rastenyte D, Birkenhäger WH *et al.* for the Systolic Hypertension in Europe (Syst-Eur) Trial Investigators. Effects of calcium channel blockade in older patients with diabetes and systolic hypertension. N Engl J Med 1999; 340: 677–684.

41. Protocol for prospective collaborative overviews of major randomized trials of blood-pressure-lowering treatments. World Health Organization/International Society of Hypertension Blood Pressure Lowering Treatment Trialists' Collaboration. J Hypertens 1998; 16: 127–137.

42. Hansson L, Lindholm LH, Niskanen L *et al.* for the Captopril Prevention Project (CAPPP) Study Group. Effect of angiotensin-converting-enzyme inhibition compared with conventional therapy on cardiovascular morbidity and mortality in hypertension: The Captopril Prevention Project randomised trial. Lancet 1999; 353: 611–616.

43. Lever AF, Hole DJ, Gillis CR *et al.* Do inhibitors of angiotensin-I-converting enzyme protect against risk of cancer? Lancet 1998; 352: 179–184.

44. Zanchetti A. Evaluating the bene-

fits of an antihypertensive agent using trials based on event and organ damage: The Systolic Hypertension in the Elderly Long-term Lacidipine (SHELL) Trial and the European Lacidipine Study on Atherosclerosis (ELSA) Trial. J Hypertens 1995; 13 (suppl 4): S35–S39.

45. Gottlieb SS, McCarter RJ, Vogel RA. Effect of beta-blockade on mortality among high-risk and low-risk patients after myocardial infarction. N Engl J Med 1998; 339: 489–497.

46. Jones JK, Gorkin L, Lian JF *et al.* Discontinuation of and changes in treatment after start of new courses of antihypertensive drugs: a study of a United Kingdom population. BMJ 1995; 311: 293–296.

47. Levine M. Costs associated with noncompliance. In: Leenen FHH, ed. Patient Compliance and the Long-Term Management of Hypertension. Montreal, Quebec: STA Communications, Canada: 1996, 21–28.

48. Bodenheimer T. The American health care system: the movement for improved quality in health care. N Engl J Med 1999; 340: 488–492.

49. Epstein AM. Rolling down the runway: the challenges ahead for quality report cards. JAMA 1998; 279: 1691–1696.

50. National Committee for Quality Assurance (NCQA). HEDIS 3.0, Vol 1. Washington, DC: National Committee for Quality Assurance, 1997.

51. Institute of Medicine. Healthy People 2000: Citizens Chart the Course. Washington, DC, USA: National Academy Press, 1990.

52. Black HR, Yi JY. A new classification for hypertension, based on relative and absolute risk, with implications for treatment and reimbursement. Hypertension 1996; 26: 719–724.

53. Neaton JD, Grimm RH Jr, Prineas RJ *et al.* Treatment of Mild Hypertension Study: final results. JAMA 1993; 270: 713–724.

54. Materson BJ, Reda DJ, Cushman WC *et al.* Single-drug therapy for hypertension in men: a comparison of six antihypertensive agents with placebo. N Engl J Med 1993; 328: 914–921.

55. Bauer JH, Reams GP. The angiotensin II type 1 receptor antagonists: a new class of antihypertensive drugs. Arch Intern Med 1995; 155: 1361–1368.

56. Bloom BS. Continuation of initial antihypertensive medication after one year. Clin Ther 1998; 20: 1–11.

2
The value of lifestyle in the management of hypertension

Lawrence J Beilin

Introduction

Maintenance of a healthy lifestyle has become recognized as one of the cornerstones of management of hypertension, alongside antihypertensive drug medication. Both the Joint National Committee of the United States and guidelines produced by the World Health Organization and the International Society of Hypertension now recommend dietary and lifestyle changes as first-line management for subjects with high normal blood pressure and for those with mild hypertension.[1,2] Lifestyle measures are also recommended as an adjunct to drug treatment in more severe grades of hypertension. These recommendations have come about as a result of a large body of evidence indicating that lifestyle factors are both major determinants of blood pressure elevation and influence the risk of cardiovascular disease independent of blood pressure. The importance of improvements in lifestyle is further emphasized by the fact that anti-hypertensive drug therapy alone fails to prevent at least 75% of cases of coronary heart disease in those with hypertension.[3] Furthermore, hypertensive patients carry a substantial burden in terms of costs, inconvenience, and side effects of medications. Moreover, the majority of patients do not achieve target blood pressures with drug therapy and only a minority are controlled on one drug alone.

It is important to consider potential benefits of lifestyle management in terms of overall cardiovascular risk and not simply in terms of blood pressure reduction. Hypertensives in countries with high levels of saturated fat consumption have a particularly high incidence of coronary heart disease.[4] In contrast, in Japan and China, where saturated fat intake has traditionally been low, stroke is the predominant cause of death in treated hypertensives.[5] The significance of this is also illustrated by mild hypertensives who smoke cigarettes, in whom quitting smoking is likely to be the single most important factor in reducing their risk of cardiovascular disease.[6] Thus, lifestyle recommendations need to be tailored according to the behavioural patterns both of individuals and the societies in which they live.

Evidence for a dominant effect of lifestyle on hypertension comes from cross-sectional and prospective population studies, from studies of migrants, and from randomized, controlled trials of the effects of changing specific dietary or other behaviours on blood pressure levels.[7] Although there is a very high incidence of hypertension in industrialized populations, the prevalence of hypertension is relatively low among those who remain slim and physically active, who drink relatively little alcohol, or who follow vegetarian dietary patterns. Thus, whereas genetic factors are critical in determining individual susceptibility to blood pressure elevation, the overall prevalence of hypertension in a community is determined by lifestyle factors interacting with multiple blood pressure regulating genes. It is worth considering the relative importance of some of the major lifestyle factors as a basis for determining priorities for patient care.

Excess body fat and physical activity

Excess body fat is the single most important factor predisposing to hypertension world-wide.[8] The relationship between increased body fat, blood pressure levels, and the prevalence of hypertension has been seen in virtually all populations that have been studied. The relationship is linear throughout the entire range of body fat and is not just a matter for the morbidly obese. The effect can be seen from infants through to the aged. Overweight or obese adolescents are more prone to hypertension in adult life. In the wealthiest nations, the majority of adults over the age of 45 years are overweight or obese, and this factor alone has been estimated to contribute around 60% of the prevalence of hypertension.[9] The incidence of obesity is increasing world-wide and it is likely that the incidence of hypertension will follow. Abdominal fat mass is most strongly related to elevated blood pressure. This form of fat distribution appears to be responsible for the so-called metabolic syndrome of dyslipidaemia, insulin resistance and hypertension.[10] Obesity also predisposes to cardiovascular disease by factors such as impaired endothelial function, increased thrombotic tendency, reduced fibrinolysis, and left ventricular hypertrophy.

Controlled trials of weight reduction show that blood pressure falls within 2–4 weeks of restricting calorie intake, with further falls as weight is lost and then stabilized. Weight loss of 4–5 kg reduces blood pressure and drug requirements in hypertensives. In mild hypertension, blood pressure falls have averaged around 1 mmHg per kilogram of weight lost. However, these falls have been doubled in some studies in which weight reduction has been combined with other lifestyle changes.

Longer-term controlled trials of weight loss programmes have shown that effects on blood pressure can be maintained over periods of 1–4 years after initial intense counselling.[11] In the USA, the TOHP1 study showed that weight control prevented the development of hypertension in a significant proportion of subjects with high normal blood pressure.[12] More recently, the TONE study demonstrated that weight control allowed antihypertensive drug therapy to be withdrawn safely in a significant proportion of older hypertensives with good blood pressure control.[13]

An increasingly sedentary lifestyle is thought to be a critical factor accounting for the rising incidence of obesity in many societies. However, it is difficult to achieve significant weight loss without initial calorie restriction in overweight hypertensives. Concomitant physical activity programmes then seem to make it easier to sustain weight control in the long term.[14]

Physical inactivity and poor physical fitness independently predispose to hypertension, diabetes mellitus, and cardiovascular disease.[15] Tackling the issue of an increasingly sedentary lifestyle is therefore a major priority for public health programmes.

In population studies, physical fitness is generally inversely related to blood pressure levels.[16] It has been difficult to evaluate the effects of physical activity on blood pressure independent of weight loss because of the lack of adequate control for confounding factors in most of the intervention trials. Overviews of the better randomized, controlled trials suggest that in previously sedentary hypertensives, physical activity equating to 40 minutes cycling three times a week at 60–70% of the maximum volume of oxygen consumption can lower systolic blood pressure by around 7 mmHg.[17] Even this level of exercise is not sustainable by many people. However, there is also evidence that less vigorous but regular activity equating to brisk walking for a total of around 40 minutes a day can reduce blood pressure to a similar extent, while at the same time substantially reducing overall cardiovascular risk.[18,19] Regular exercise may be of particular value for hypertensives with non-insulin-dependent diabetes, in whom physical training can improve glucose tolerance as well as aiding weight control and improving endothelial dysfunction.[20] Health recommendations generally emphasize aerobic activity in subjects with established hypertension because there is concern that intense weight-bearing or isometric exercise may be hazardous by virtue of excessive rises in blood pressure and cardiac stress.

Current recommendations are therefore to encourage people to increase leisure time and incidental activity by frequent walks, climbing stairs, and so on, with the addition of jogging, swimming, cycling, light weight-bearing aerobics, and other leisure pursuits when opportune. These efforts need to start in schools because the problems of overweight and inactivity are increasingly prevalent in young schoolchildren and adolescents.[21,22]

Dietary changes

Salt and potassium

Over recent decades, dietary salt intake has received more attention than other lifestyle factors in relation to predisposition to hypertension. However, it is now recognized as being only one of a number of dietary constituents that affect blood pressure levels. The average sodium intake of most communities exceeds physiologic requirements by a factor of between 10 and 20. There is still some controversy about the importance of sodium chloride in determining blood pressure levels in the general population.[23–25] Much of this controversy is due to difficulty in accurately assessing individuals' usual salt intake. In an overview of the epidemiologic and clinical trial data, Law reanalysed population data taking into account measurement errors,[26] and estimated that a reduction in sodium intake by 50 mmol a day would decrease systolic blood pressure in people aged over 50 years by about 5 mmHg and could reduce coronary deaths in the UK by around 16% per year and age-specific stroke mortality by 22%.

Not all people are sensitive to the pressor effects of salt and concern has been expressed that sodium restriction may have adverse effects in terms of lipid profile and increases in plasma renin and angiotensin synthesis. Adverse changes in lipids have been seen only in very short-term studies with extremes of sodium restriction (down to 10–20 mmol per day).[27] They do not occur with the more moderate levels of sodium restriction that have been shown to reduce blood pressure in hypertensives.[28,29]

It has also been argued that severe sodium restriction would impose an unnecessary burden on the population and create problems in food manufacture. However, since the average sodium intake in countries such as the USA is still around 180 mmol per day in men, with up to half the population consuming up to 300 mmol per day, a reduction by up to 100 mmol per day is not extreme. In many instances this could be achieved by avoiding added salt and high-salt processed foods and by minimizing the use of salt in cooking. However, the major part of sodium intake nowadays comes from food and to achieve intakes between 70 and 100 mmol per day requires greater availability of low-salt bread, spreads, and meat products and the use of salt substitutes.

In the case of subjects with established hypertension, the case is more clear-cut. Falls in systolic blood pressure of around 6 mmHg have been achieved when sodium intake is reduced to around 80 mmol per day in randomized placebo-controlled trials.[30] The effect is dose-dependent and is proportional to the height of the blood pressure.[31,32] Most of the trials of salt restriction have been of only a few weeks' duration. However, some evidence for the efficacy and safety of prolonged reduction in sodium intake was shown in the recent TONE study in older hypertensives.[13] This

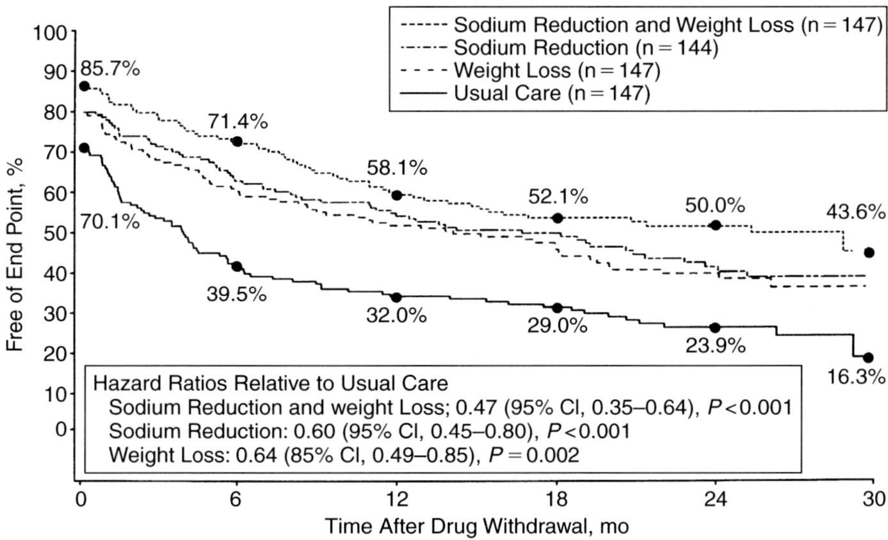

Figure 2.1

The TONE study. Percentages of the 144 participants assigned to reduced sodium intake, the 147 assigned to weight loss, the 147 assigned to reduced sodium intake and weight loss combined, and the 147 assigned to usual care (no lifestyle intervention) who remained free of cardiovascular events and high blood pressure and did not have an antihypertensive agent prescribed during follow-up. From Whelton *et al.* JAMA 1998; 279: 839–846, with permission. Copyrighted 1998 American Medical Association.

trial also showed an additive effect of salt reduction and weight loss. In this trial, older hypertensives with well-controlled blood pressure were entered in a phase of withdrawal of drug therapy after 3 months of intense dietary counselling. They were randomized to sodium restriction or weight loss if obese, or to both measures combined. Significantly more of those on the dietary regimes were able to remain off drug therapy and they had fewer cardiovascular events after an average 29 months follow-up. The group that combined weight loss with sodium restriction showed the greatest success rate (*Fig. 2.1*). Interestingly, sodium intake fell by only 40 mmol per day on average, again illustrating that in older hypertensives modest reduction in excess salt intake improves blood pressure control.

Evidence that sodium restriction may help to prevent hypertension comes from the TOHP1 study in subjects with high normal pressures.[12] Those who were offered a salt restriction regime for 3 years were less likely than controls to develop blood pressure over 140/90 mmHg despite average reductions in salt intake of less than 30 mmol per day. Other trials have shown dose–response effects in older hypertensives when sodium intake has been reduced by 50 or 100 mmol per day in a double-blind fashion.

Effects of most antihypertensive drug groups can be enhanced by sodium restriction, thereby offering the opportunity of improving blood pressure control and minimizing drug use. Given the decreasing use of diuretics in hypertension and the relatively poor blood pressure control achieved in the majority of patients in general practice, avoidance of excessive salt consumption should be given higher priority along with other lifestyle measures in hypertensive patients.

Intake of dietary potassium tends to be inversely related to salt consumption, and there is evidence suggesting that the pressor effects of sodium are exacerbated when potassium consumption is low.[33,34] Dietary potassium intake has also been associated with lower stroke rates in population studies.[35] However, these phenomena may be confounded by the strong association between different dietary and lifestyle habits. For example, potassium is found in high concentrations in fruit and vegetables, which may contain other constituents that both predispose to blood pressure reduction and protect against vascular disease. Nevertheless, randomized controlled trials of 40–60 mmol per day of potassium supplements in hypertensives have shown systolic blood pressure falls of around 4 mmHg.[36] However, for reasons described below, it seems advisable to increase potassium intake via potassium-rich foods rather than by supplements.

Complex dietary changes

People eat foods and not individual nutrients and it should not be so surprising that more complex food patterns than those described above should be associated with effects on blood pressure. Populations that adhere to strict ovolactovegetarian or vegan eating habits have lower blood pressures and less hypertension than their meat-eating counterparts.[37] Such populations often have a strong religious base and eschew the use of alcohol, tobacco and caffeine. In an elegant comparison of Seventh Day Adventist ovolactovegetarians with meat-eating Mormons, Rouse *et al.* were able to demonstrate that systolic blood pressure was about 5 mmHg lower in the vegetarians independent of effects of obesity and other lifestyle differences.[38] The vegetarians also had one-fifth of the prevalence of mild hypertension compared with the meat eaters. In subsequent randomized, controlled trials, regular meat eaters were given diets similar in composition to those eaten by the Adventist vegetarians. Both normotensives and untreated hypertensives showed blood pressure falls of around 6/3 mmHg over periods of 6 weeks. These effects were independent of small changes in weight or dietary sodium or potassium, and they were reversible when the usual diet was resumed.[39,40]

In addition to the avoidance of meat, poultry and fish, the vegetarian diets in these studies were characterized by increased amounts of fruit, vegetables, high-fibre cereals, and bread and by relative increases in polyunsaturated fats over saturated fats.

Subsequent dietary trials have suggested that the blood-pressure-lowering effects of the vegetarian diets were due neither to the absence of meat products nor to any specific food component but to the complex dietary patterns.[40–42]

This conclusion has been confirmed in the recent Dietary Approach to Stopping Hypertension (DASH) study in which subjects with normal blood pressure or mild hypertension were randomized to either increase fruit and vegetable consumption to 5 serves a day or, in addition, to substitute saturated fats for low-fat dairy products over an 8-week period.[43] Lean meat, poultry, and fish consumption were encouraged with the combination diet. Increasing fruit and vegetable consumption alone led to blood pressure falls averaging 2.8/1.1 mmHg, whereas the group that also changed fat intake showed a further fall in blood pressure by 5.5/3.0 mmHg. The subgroup of mild hypertensives showed the greatest blood pressure fall, averaging 11.4/5.5 mmHg compared with controls. Factors in the fruit and vegetable diet that may act in concert to lower blood pressure include potassium, magnesium, fibre, and antioxidants.

Diets of this nature are likely to be acceptable by a wider section of the community than strict vegetarian diets. They also have better nutrient value. The combination diet also has the potential to reduce overall cardiovascular risk by reducing low-density lipoprotein cholesterol levels. Body weight and dietary salt intake changed little in DASH and it will be interesting to see whether there is any additional influence of weight loss or sodium restriction with these complex dietary changes in the longer term.

Fish

Increased consumption of dietary long-chain polyunsaturated n-3 fatty acids in fish may help reduce blood pressure levels in hypertensives.[44] These n-3 fatty acids have several other important biological actions that may reduce the risk of atherothrombotic disease. These effects include:

(a) reducing platelet aggregation;
(b) decreasing serum triglyceride levels;
(c) increasing high-density lipoprotein-2 cholesterol levels;
(d) improving endothelial dilator function;
(e) decreasing heart rate and myocardial excitability; and
(f)   decreasing inflammatory responses.[45]

Randomized controlled trials of fish oil supplements that contain mixtures of 5–6 g per day of the n-3 fatty acids eicosapentanoic acid and docosahexanoic acid have shown systolic blood pressure reductions of around 6 mmHg in untreated hypertensives[44,45] and in hypertensives with type 2 diabetes.[46] Studies from Perth in Western Australia have shown that eating a daily fish meal that contains about 3.6 g per day of n-3 fatty acids has similar effects on lipids and platelet function to those of comparable doses of fish oils in dyslipidaemic subjects.[47]

In a recent factorial study in overweight hypertensives, a daily fish meal and a weight-reducing regime were shown to have independent and additive effects on blood pressure reduction. Incorporating a daily fish meal into a weight-reducing regime led to blood pressure falls of 13/9 mmHg in daytime ambulatory blood pressure compared with controls.[48] The combination diet also led to the greatest falls in triglycerides and maximum improvements in glucose tolerance.[49] Together, these changes could substantially reduce the risk of cardiovascular disease. Additional benefits are likely to accrue from effects of n-3 fatty acids on platelet, endothelial, and myocardial function. The quantities of fish required to achieve these effects ranged from 60 to 200 g per day, depending on the n-3 fatty acid content of the fish, and they could easily be obtained as fresh or canned products.

When these data are combined with epidemiological and clinical trial evidence for a protective effect of marine oils on coronary events, there is a good case for recommending increased fish consumption as part of a healthy diet for hypertensives. Rather than taking fish oil supplements, replacing some meat with fish has the advantage that it is more likely to lead to a reduction in saturated fat intake and total calories derived from fat.

Other aspects of lifestyle

Alcohol consumption

In drinking populations, alcohol consumption is statistically second only to obesity as a major factor predisposing to hypertension.[50] The effect of alcohol on blood pressure appears to increase linearly with increasing levels of consumption.[51,52] People who drink three or more standard drinks a day have a 2-fold to 3-fold increased prevalence of mild hypertension compared with those who drink up to one drink a day. The effect of alcohol on blood pressure is seen in all major ethnic groups, in both men and women, and with all types of alcoholic beverage.[53] The effect appears to be greater with ageing but has been described in adolescents. The effect may be greater in smokers and is additive to the effects of obesity. The effects of alcohol on blood pressure are partially reversible over 3–4 weeks of alcohol moderation. In heavy drinkers, some of the effect may be mediated by acute alcohol withdrawal following heavy weekend drinking.[54,55]

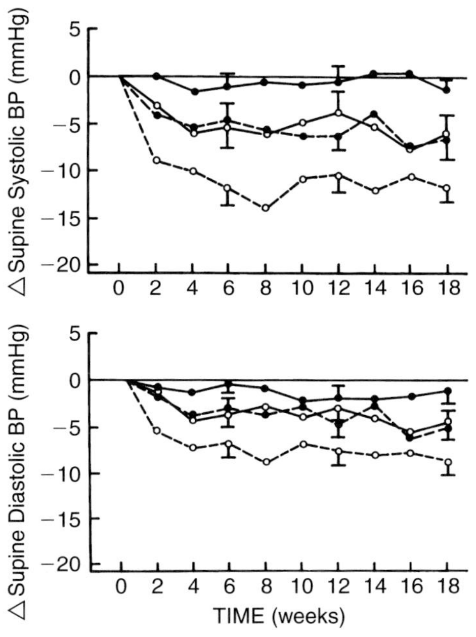

Figure 2.2

Change in group mean (and standard error of the mean) systolic and diastolic blood pressures (BP) in the four study groups in a study by Puddey *et al.*, 1992.[58] Used with permission.

●——● Normal alcohol intake, normal caloric intake (n = 20)
●– – –● Normal alcohol intake, low caloric intake (n = 22)
○——○ Low alcohol intake, normal caloric intake (n = 21)
○– – –○ Low alcohol intake, low caloric intake (n = 23)

Drinking alcohol can increase antihypertensive drug requirements. Problem drinkers are more likely to present with resistant hypertension owing to poor compliance with drug therapy.

Randomized, controlled trials that have involved drinkers changing from normal alcoholic beverages to very low alcohol beers have shown falls in blood pressure in patients with treated and untreated mild hypertension of around 1 mmHg for each standard drink per day reduction.[56,57] Larger effects are likely with severe hypertension and in heavier drinkers.

In a factorial study from Perth in Western Australia, simultaneous reduction of weight and alcohol consumption in overweight subjects with mild hypertension resulted in blood pressure falls that average 10–14 mmHg systolic and 9 mmHg diastolic over 4 months.[58] Effects of weight control and alcohol moderation were additive (*Fig. 2.2*) and led to maximum improvement in lipid profile and in left ventricular function.

The effects of alcohol on cardiovascular morbidity and mortality are complex.[59] At lower levels of consumption there is up to 20% protection against coronary events in populations prone to coronary artery disease. There may also be some protection against ischaemic stroke in those drinking up to three standard drinks a day.[60] However, the risk of haemorrhagic stroke appears to increase progressively throughout the range of consumption.[61] Heavier drinking and binge drinking patterns are associated with increased risk of both haemorrhagic and ischaemic stroke, cardiomyopathy, and cardiac arrhythmias. Population guidelines clearly need to consider all physical and psychosocial aspects of drinking.[62] Current advice to hypertensive drinkers is to limit consumption to no more than two standard drinks a day for men and one for women.

There has been much publicity concerning the so-called French paradox and the hypothesis that red wine may have more cardioprotective effects than other types of beverage. However, lower rates of coronary heart disease have been seen with all types of alcohol beverage in different countries and are probably mediated by effects of ethanol *per se* increasing high-density lipoprotein cholesterol and reducing platelet aggregation.[63] Drinkers of wine, spirits, and beer often have quite different lifestyle characteristics from one another, which are likely to have an impact on their risk of cardiovascular disease. Such cultural dietary and lifestyle factors are more likely to account for low rates of coronary heart disease in France.

Smoking

Smoking cigarettes increases the risk of coronary deaths by a factor of about three in subjects with hypertension in countries with Western-type diets. It seems that stopping smoking largely reverses this risk over a period of 3–5 years.[64,65] Thus, when the main cause of death is likely to be coronary heart disease the benefits of smoking cessation are substantially greater than, but complementary to, the effects of antihypertensive drug therapy.

The effects of smoking on blood pressure *per se* are less clear. Smoking a cigarette elevates blood pressure acutely for 10–15 minutes. This effect may be prolonged for up to 2 hours if combined with a strong cup of coffee.[66] However, smokers' resting blood pressure as measured in the clinic in epidemiological studies tends to be lower than that of non-smokers.[51] This is partly but not entirely accounted for by the fact that smokers tend to be less obese. Data from ambulatory blood pressure measurements may help to explain this paradox: several studies suggest that in people who smoke regularly during the day, blood pressures are higher than non-smokers, whereas comparison of ambulatory and clinic blood pressures suggest that the blood pressure of smokers may be less subject to a 'white coat' effect.[67]

Regardless of these nuances, the health benefits of stopping smoking in hypertensives are deemed to be such as to make this the highest priority in lifestyle management. Such advice will need to be accompanied by measures to avoid the weight gain that often follows cessation of smoking and that may lead to an increase rather than a decrease in blood pressure.

Caffeine consumption

Caffeine-containing beverages such as tea and coffee can cause acute elevations of blood pressure of 5–15 mmHg systolic. The effects are usually over within 1 hour unless combined with smoking. The effects of these beverages on long-term blood pressure regulation have been less clear, but there is some evidence from controlled trials that drinking four or five cups of coffee a day may increase ambulatory systolic blood pressures by around 6 mmHg, particularly in older patients with hypertension.[68] Such patients should be advised either to avoid a high intake of coffee or to take decaffeinated beverages.

Stress

Whereas the acute pressor effects of psychological stress on blood pressure are clear-cut, effects on long-term blood pressure regulation are uncertain. There are major methodological problems in defining stress and stressors.[69] Very often what is perceived as stressful by an external observer is not recognized as such by the subject. Pickering's group in New York have used Karacek's model of job strain, in which perceived work stress is coupled with inability of the individual to control the situation. They have provided some evidence that men with high job strain have the highest blood pressures, particularly if they drink alcohol.[70] Increases in blood pressure over a 3-year period were also greatest in those with high job strain.[71]

Job strain tends to be related to a number of behaviours that may themselves raise blood pressure, and it is often difficult to correct adequately for such confounding influences. In a study on Australian Tax Department workers, Lindquist *et al.* found no relationship between resting blood pressure and perceived job stress.[72] However, maladaptive strategies used to cope with stress, such as heavier drinking, smoking, and poor eating habits, were related to blood pressure. They concluded from their study that the effects of job or home stress on blood pressure were more likely to be related to the nature of the lifestyle coping strategies used by the individual. Interestingly, women generally used healthier coping strategies than men to cope with stress.

Certain personality types appear more prone to develop hypertension. This seems to apply particularly to people who have 'suppressed hostility' or difficulty in expressing their emotions. Again, it is unclear whether or not the effects on blood pressure are due to intrinsic differences in blood pressure regulation in such subjects or whether they are mediated by drinking, eating, or physical activity habits.

There have been a number of attempts to use stress management techniques of various kinds to lower blood pressure in hypertensives. Very few studies have been adequately controlled and adjusted for potential confounding influences.[73] The better studies have generally been negative or have shown marginal benefit. People can be taught to relax at the time of blood pressure measurement but it has yet to be demonstrated whether this converts to more effective 24-hour blood pressure control when subjects are unaware that their blood pressure is being recorded. Changing lifelong ingrained habits is difficult, particularly in the face of home and workplace stress, so in this respect stress management techniques may be required to help hypertensives and others at high risk of cardiovascular disease to achieve and maintain some of the lifestyle changes being recommended.

Conclusions

From the above, it can be seen that there are a number of lifestyle changes that may help hypertensive patients to minimize drug requirements and reduce the risk of cardiovascular events. For those with borderline and mild hypertension, it may be safe to introduce such measures and persist over several months so that those able to reverse the disorder of blood pressure regulation can do so without needing to depend on lifelong drug therapy. However, lifelong monitoring is advisable for all hypertensives given the propensity for lost weight to be regained and unhealthy drinking or eating habits to be resumed.

In the case of those already on drug therapy and who have well-controlled blood pressure on one or two drugs, it may be possible to withdraw therapy cautiously following demonstrable and sustained lifestyle changes. Regular and continued monitoring of blood pressure is essential, since it has been shown that without lifestyle change, blood pressure may stay down initially on cessation of drugs but will inevitably rise over the next 3–4 years.

For the majority of hypertensives who continue to require drugs, lifestyle changes have the capacity not only to minimize drug requirements but may also offer a range of options for diminishing the risk of cardiovascular disease independent of effects on blood pressure. This is particularly so with smoking cessation, avoidance of obesity, increased physical activity, moderation of heavy alcohol and high salt consumption, reduction in saturated fat intake, and increased consumption of fruit, vegetables, fish, and low-fat dairy products. In most cases, the potential health benefits also extend well beyond prevention of cardiovascular disease.

One of the biggest difficulties facing the medical profession is how to help patients to achieve lifestyle changes. Intrinsic scepticism by the profession as to the effectiveness of such changes or the ability of their patients to modify lifestyle is a major obstacle in itself. However, the growing body of evidence of the substantial reversibility of hypertension and the importance of associated lifestyle-dependent cardiovascular risk factors has led to incorporation of the above ideas into national and international guidelines for hypertension management. The critical role of the doctor or allied health professional in assisting a significant proportion of smokers to stop or heavier drinkers to moderate their intake is now accepted as the norm. The success rate for these and other lifestyle changes is still far too low, but it can be improved by using well-tested behavioural modification techniques. However, patient counselling and education need time and training no less than do methods to improve patient compliance with drug therapy.

Over and above the individual approach is the need for well-designed public health campaigns that both inform patients and enable them to distinguish recommendations based on firm scientific evidence from the many panaceas on offer by the health-food industry.

Changes in eating patterns need to be facilitated by the food industry, with encouragement and, where necessary, legislation to ensure proper food labelling and availability of healthier products.

Hypertension and its consequences is already of major importance in industrialized nations, in many of which over half of the population over the age of 60 years are receiving antihypertensive drug therapy. It has been estimated that in the coming decades this will be one of the major problems worldwide as developing countries overcome infectious disease and adopt a Western lifestyle. In these circumstances, lifestyles that minimize the risk of hypertensive cardiovascular disease will be of crucial economic importance.

References

1. The Sixth Report of the Joint National Committee on Prevention, Detection, Evaluation and Treatment of High Blood Pressure. Arch Intern Med 1997; 157: 2413–2446.

2. Guidelines Subcommittee. 1999 World Health Organization–International Society of Hypertension Guidelines for the Management of Hypertension Guidelines Subcommittee. J Hypertens 1999; 17: 151–183.

3. Collins R, MacMahon S. Blood pressure, antihypertensive treatment and the risks of stroke and coronary heart disease. Br Med Bull 1994; 52: 272–298.

4. Wilson PW, D'Agostino RB, Levy D et al. Prediction of coronary heart disease using risk factor categories. Circulation 1998; 97: 1837–1847.

5. Marmot MG, Syme SL, Kagon A et al. Epidemiologic studies of coronary heart disease and stroke in Japanese now living in Japan, Hawaii and California: prevalence of coronary and hypertensive heart disease and associated risk factors. Am J Epidemiol 1975; 102: 514–525.

6. Medical Research Council Working Party. MRC trial of treatment of mild hypertension: principal results. BMJ 1985; 291: 97–104.

7. Beilin LJ. The Fifth Sir George Pickering Memorial Lecture. Epitaph to essential hypertension: a preventable disorder of known aetiology (editorial review)? J Hypertens 1988; 6: 85–94.

8. Stamler J. Epidemiologic findings on body mass and blood pressure in adults. Ann Epidemiol 1991; 1: 347–362.

9. MacMahon S, Cutler J, Brittain E, Higgins M. Obesity and hypertension: epidemiological and clinical issues. Eur Heart J 1987; 8: 57–70.

10. Pouliot MC, Despres JP, Lemieux S *et al.* Waist circumference and abdominal sagittal diameter: best single anthropometric indexes of abdominal visceral adipose tissue accumulation and related cardiovascular risk in men and women. Am J Cardiol 1994; 73: 460–468.

11. Stamler R, Stamler J, Gosch FS *et al.* Primary prevention of hypertension by nutritional hygienic means: final report of a randomized controlled trial. JAMA 1989; 262: 1801–1807.

12. TOHP I: The Trials of Hypertension Prevention Collaborative Research Group. Effect of weight loss and sodium reduction intervention on blood pressure and hypertension incidence in overweight people with high normal blood pressure: the Trials of Hypertension Prevention, phase II. Arch Intern Med 1997; 157: 657–667.

13. Whelton PK, Appel LJ, Espeland MA *et al.* Tone Collaborative Research Group. Sodium reduction and weight loss in the treatment of hypertension in older persons. A randomized controlled Trial of Nonpharmacologic Interventions in the Elderly (TONE). JAMA 1998; 279: 839–846.

14. Blair SN. Evidence for success of exercise in weight loss and control. Ann Intern Med 1993; 119: 702–706.

15. Paffenbarger RS Jr, Hyde RT, Wing AL *et al.* The association of changes in physical activity level and other lifestyle characteristics with mortality among men. N Engl J Med 1993; 328: 538–545.

16. Blair SN, Goodyear NN, Gibbons LW, Cooper KH. Physical fitness and incidence of hypertension in healthy normotensive men and women. JAMA 1984; 252: 487–490.

17. Fagard RH. The role of exercise in blood pressure control: supportive evidence. J Hypertens 1995; 13: 1223–1227.

18. Jennings GLR. Exercise and blood pressure: walk, run or swim? J Hypertens 1997; 15: 567–569.

19. US Department of Health and Human Services. Physical activity and health: a report of the Surgeon General. Atlanta, Georgia, USA: Centers for Disease Control and Prevention and Health Promotion, 1996.

20. Dunstan DW, Mori TA, Puddey IB *et al.* The independent and combined effects of aerobic exercise and dietary fish on serum lipids and glycemic control in non-insulin-dependent diabetes mellitus. A randomized controlled study. Diabetes Care 1997; 20: 913–921.

21. Berenson GS, Wattigney WA, Bao W *et al.* Epidemiology of early primary hypertension and implications for prevention: the Bogalusa Heart Study. J Hum Hypertens 1994; 8: 303–311.

22. Burke V, Milligan RAK, Beilin LJ *et al.* Clustering of health-related behaviors in 18-year-old Australians. Prev Med 1997; 26: 724–733.

23. Stamler R. Implications of the INTERSALT Study. Hypertens

1991; 17 (suppl 1): I-16–I-20.

24. Alderman MH, Anderson S, Bennett WM *et al.* Nutrition Science Policy: scientists' statement regarding data on the sodium–hypertension relationship and sodium health claims on food labelling. Nutr Rev 1997; 55: 172–175.

25. Kunanyika S, Cutler JA. Dietary sodium reduction: is there a cause for concern? J Am Coll Nutr 1997; 16: 192–203.

26. Law MR. Epidemiological evidence on salt and blood pressure. Am J Hypertens 1997; 10 (suppl 5): 42S–45S.

27. Del Rio A, Rodriquez-Villamil JL. Metabolic effects of strict salt restriction in essential hypertensive patients. J Intern Med 1993; 233: 409–414.

28. Sciarrone SEG, Beilin LJ, Rouse IL, Rogers PB. A factorial study of salt restriction and a low-fat/high fiber diet in hypertensive subjects. J Hypertens 1992; 10: 287–298.

29. Meland A, Laerum E, Aakvaag A *et al.* Salt restriction: effects on lipids and insulin production in hypertensive patients. Scand J Clin Lab Invest 1995; 57: 501–505.

30. Cutler JA, Follman D, Alexander PS. Randomized controlled trials of sodium reduction: an overview. Am J Clin Nutr 1997; 65 (suppl): 643S–651S.

31. MacGregor GA, Markandu ND, Sagnella GA *et al.* Double-blind study of three sodium intakes and long term effects of sodium restriction in essential hypertension. Lancet 1989; ii: 1244–1247.

32. Cappuccio FP, Markandu ND, Carney C *et al.* Double-blind study of modest salt restriction in older people. Lancet 1997; 350: 850–854.

33. Stamler J. The Intersalt Study: background, methods, findings and implications. Am J Clin Nutr 1997; 65 (suppl): 626S–642S.

34. Khaw KT, Barrett-Connor E. Dietary potassium and blood pressure in a population. Am J Clin Nutr 1984; 39: 963–968.

35. Stamler J, Elliott P, Kesteloot H *et al.* Inverse relation of dietary protein markers with blood pressure. Circulation 1996; 94: 1629–1634.

36. Whelton PK, He J, Cutler JA *et al.* Effects of oral potassium on blood pressure: meta-analysis of randomized controlled trials. JAMA 1997; 277: 1624–1632.

37. Burke V, Beilin LJ, Sciarrone S. Vegetarian diets, protein and fiber. Part 3: pathogenesis. In: Swales JD, ed. Textbook of Hypertension. London: Blackwell Scientific Publications, 1994, 619–632.

38. Rouse IL, Armstrong BK, Beilin LJ. The relationship of blood pressure to diet and lifestyle in two religious populations. J Hypertens 1983; 1: 65–71.

39. Rouse IL, Beilin LJ, Armstrong BK, Vandongen R. Blood pressure lowering effect of a vegetarian diet: a controlled trial in normotensive subjects. Lancet 1983; i: 5–10.

40. Margetts BM, Beilin LJ, Vandongen R, Armstrong BK. Vegetarian diet in mild hypertension: a randomized controlled trial. BMJ 1986; 293: 1468–1471.

41. Kestin M, Rouse IL, Correll RA, Nestel PJ. Cardiovascular disease risk factors in free-living men: comparisons of two prudent diets, one based on lacto-ovo-vegetarianism and the other allowing lean meat. Am J Clin Nutr 1989; 50: 280–287.

42. Prescott SL, Jenner DA, Beilin LJ *et al.* A randomized controlled trial of the effect on blood pressure of dietary non-meat protein

versus meat protein in normotensive omnivores. Clin Sci 1988; 74: 665–672.

43. Appel LJ, Morre TJ, Obarzanetk E *et al.* A clinical trial of the effects of dietary patterns on blood pressure. DASH Collaborative Research Group. N Engl J Med 1997; 336: 1117–1124.

44. Appel LJ, Miller ER III, Seidler AJ, Whelton PK. Does supplementation of diet with 'fish oil' reduce blood pressure? Arch Intern Med 1993; 53: 1429–1438.

45. Stone NJ. Fish consumption, fish oil, lipids, and coronary heart disease. Am J Clin Nutr 1997; 65: 1083–1086.

46. Grundt H, Nilsen DWT, Hetland O *et al.* Improvement of serum lipids and blood pressure during intervention with n-3 fatty acids was not associated with changes in insulin levels in subjects with combined hyperlipidaemia. J Intern Med 1995; 237: 249–259.

47. Vandongen R, Mori TA, Burke V *et al.* Effects on blood pressure of omega-3 fats in subjects at increased risk of cardiovascular disease. Hypertension 1993; 22: 371–379.

48. Bao DQ, Mori TA, Burke V *et al.* Effects of dietary fish and weight reduction on ambulatory blood pressure in overweight hypertensives. Hypertension 1998; 32: 710–717.

49. Mori TA, Bao DQ, Burke V *et al.* Dietary fish as a major component of a weight reducing diet: impact on serum lipids, glucose and insulin metabolism in overweight hypertensive subjects. Am J Clin Nutr; in press.

50. Puddey IB, Beilin LJ, Rakic V. Alcohol, hypertension and the cardiovascular system: a critical appraisal. Addiction Biol 1997; 2: 159–170.

51. Arkwright PD, Beilin LJ, Rouse I *et al.* Effects of alcohol use and other aspects of life-style on blood pressure levels and prevalence of hypertension in a working population. Circulation 1982; 66: 60–66.

52. Moreira LB, Fuchs FD, Moraes RS *et al.* Alcohol intake and blood pressure: the importance of time elapsed since last drink. J Hypertens 1998; 16: 175–180.

53. Klatsky A, Friedman G, Siegelaub A, Gerard M. Alcohol consumption and blood pressure. Kaiser-Permanente Multiphasic Health Examination Data. N Engl J Med 1977; 296: 1194–1200.

54. Wannamethee G, Shaper AG. Alcohol intake and variations in blood pressure by day of examination. J Hum Hypertens 1991; 5: 57–62.

55. Rakic V, Puddey IB, Burke V *et al.* Influence of pattern of alcohol intake on blood pressure in regular drinkers: a controlled trial. J Hypertens 1998; 16: 165–174.

56. Puddey IB, Beilin LJ, Vandongen R. Regular alcohol use raises blood pressure in treated hypertensive subjects: a randomized controlled trial. Lancet 1987; i: 647–650.

57. Hsieh ST, Saito K, Miyajima T *et al.* Effects of alcohol moderation on blood pressure and intracellular cations in mild essential hypertension. Am J Hypertens 1995; 8: 696–703.

58. Puddey IB, Parker M, Beilin LJ *et al.* Effects of alcohol and caloric restrictions on blood pressure and serum lipids in overweight men. Hypertension 1992; 20: 533–541.

59. Thun MJ, Peto R, Lopez AD *et al.* Alcohol consumption and mortality among middle-aged and elderly US adults. N Engl J Med 1997; 337: 1705–1714.

60. Sacco RL, Elkind M, Boden-

Albala B *et al.* The protective effect of moderate alcohol consumption on ischemic stroke. JAMA 1999; 281: 53–60.

61. Donahue RP, Abbott RD, Reed DM, Yano K. Alcohol and hemorrhagic stroke: the Honolulu Heart Program. JAMA 1986; 255: 2311–2314.

62. Jackson R, Beaglehole R. Alcohol consumption guidelines: relative safety vs absolute risks and benefits. Lancet 1995; 346: 716.

63. Law M, Wald N. Why heart disease mortality is low in France: the time lag explanation. BMJ 1999; 318: 1471–1480.

64. Kawachi J, Colditz GA, Stampfer MJ *et al.* Smoking cessation and time course of decreased risks of coronary heart disease in middle-aged women. Arch Intern Med 1994; 154: 169–175.

65. Doll R, Peto R. Mortality in relation to smoking 20 years observation on male British doctors. BMJ 1976; ii: 1525–1536.

66. Freestone S, Ramsay LE. Effect of coffee and cigarette smoking on the blood pressure of patients with accelerated (malignant) hypertension. J Hum Hypertens 1995; 9: 89–91.

67. Narkiewicz K, Maraglino G, Biason T *et al.* Interactive effect of cigarettes and coffee on daytime systolic blood pressure in patients with mild essential hypertension. HARVEST Study Group. J Hypertens 1995; 13: 965–970.

68. Rakic V, Burke V, Beilin LJ. Effects of coffee on ambulatory blood pressure in older men and women: a randomized controlled trial. Hypertension 1999; 33: 869–873.

69. Nyklicek I, Vingerhoets JJM, Van Heck GL. Hypertension and objective and self-reported stressor exposure: a review. J Psychosom Res 1996; 40: 585–601.

70. Pickering TG, Devereux RB, James GD *et al.* Environmental influences on blood pressure and the role of job strain. J Hypertens 1996; 14 (suppl 5): S179–S185.

71. Schwartz JE, Schnall PL, Pickering TG. The effect of job strain on ambulatory blood pressure in men over 6 years is comparable to other risk factors (abstract). International Society of Hypertension, Glasgow. J Hypertens 1996; 14 (suppl 1): S4.

72. Lindquist TL, Beilin LJ, Knuiman MW. Influence of lifestyle, coping and job stress on blood pressure in men and women. Hypertension 1997; 29: 1–7.

73. Eisenberg DM, Delbanco TL, Berkey CS *et al.* Cognitive behavioural techniques for hypertension. Are they effective? Ann Intern Med 1993; 118: 964–978.

3
Deciding on the need for drug therapy

Rodney Jackson

Introduction

There is a substantial evidence base demonstrating that drugs that lower blood pressure reduce the relative risk of cardiovascular disease (CVD) in patients with mildly raised blood pressure. In adults, including those over the age of 80 years, pharmacotherapy for 3–5 years reduces the combined risk of coronary and stroke events by about one-third[1,2] and shows no increase in non-cardiovascular mortality.[3] Comparable data on non-cardiovascular morbidity is not available, although trials and case–control studies suggest no increase in the incidence of cancer with antihypertensive therapy. Moreover, quality of life does not appear to be adversely affected by drug therapy.[4,5]

However, for several reasons considerable uncertainty remains about which patients should receive drug treatment. First, there is a continuous relationship between blood pressure and CVD risk down to low levels, with no obvious blood pressure treatment threshold.[6] As a result, recommended treatment thresholds vary considerably and these differences have significant effects on the numbers of patients who are eligible for treatment. Second, blood pressure alone is a poor predictor of CVD risk among patients with mildly raised blood pressure, and the presence of other CVD risk factors often has a greater impact on the absolute benefits of lowering blood pressure than the pre-treatment blood pressure itself.[7,8] Although most treatment recommendations now explicitly consider other risk factors, the approaches vary considerably and these differences also have substantial effects on patient eligibility for treatment.

The differences between recommendations are confusing for practitioners and it is not surprising there is so much variation in practice when the experts cannot agree. Since the majority of patients with mild hypertension are managed by clinical generalists, most of whom do not have the time or expertise to carry out a personal, in-depth review of the evidence, it is essential that they receive consistent, well-justified, evidence-based guidance that can be applied in busy practice settings.

The aim of this chapter is to provide clinicians with clear and consistent

evidence-based advice about which patients who have mildly raised blood pressure should be considered for treatment with blood pressure-lowering drugs. The choice of drugs is covered in later chapters. This chapter focuses on the two issues that have caused most uncertainty around treatment decisions:

(a) definitions of hypertension and blood pressure treatment thresholds; and
(b) the influence of other CVD risk factors on drug treatment decisions.

This chapter examines the four major national and international reports that provide recommendations on the management of hypertension that have been published since 1997. These reports, which have all involved extensive reviews of the relevant evidence, come from:

(a) the USA (the sixth report of the Joint National Committee on Prevention, Detection, Evaluation, and Treatment of High Blood Pressure, 1997;[9] referred to in this chapter as JNC);
(b) the United Kingdom (Joint British Recommendations on Prevention of Coronary Heart Disease in Clinical Practice, 1998;[10] referred to as British);
(c) Europe (Joint European Societies Recommendations on Prevention of Coronary Heart Disease in Clinical Practice, 1998;[11] referred to as European); and
(d) an international committee (World Health Organization–International Society of Hypertension Guidelines on the Management of Hypertension, 1998;[12] referred to as WHO–ISH).

The recommendations from each of these reports that relate specifically to definitions of hypertension, blood pressure treatment thresholds and consideration of other risk factors in treatment decisions are described and discussed. The similarities and differences between the guidelines are identified and an attempt is made to integrate their recommendations in order to provide more consistent, valid guidance for busy clinical generalists and their patients. Throughout this chapter, diastolic blood pressure levels used, refer to Phase V diastolic pressure (i.e. the disappearance of Korotkoff sounds).

Classification of blood pressure levels

The guidelines

Two of the four guidelines reviewed (JNC, WHO–ISH) provide similar, detailed classifications of blood pressure levels, which divide patients into categories of optimal, normal, and high-normal blood pressure and three stages or grades of hypertension (*Table 3.1*). The 1998 WHO–ISH report intentionally used the same major categories as the 1997 JNC

Table 3.1 Classification of blood pressure levels in the JNC VI[9] and the WHO–ISH[12] guidelines on the management of hypertension. (Note that the European and British guidelines do not provide a detailed classification of blood pressure levels.)

JNC[9]			WHO–ISH[12]		
Blood pressure category	Systolic blood pressure (mmHg)	Diastolic blood pressure (mmHg)	Blood pressure category	Systolic blood pressure (mmHg)	Diastolic blood pressure (mmHg)*
Optimal	<120	<80	Optimal	<120	<80
Normal	<130	<85	Normal	<130	<85
High-normal	130–139	85–89	High-normal	130–139	85–89
Hypertension			Hypertension		
Stage 1 (mild)	140–159	90–99	Grade 1	140–159	90–99
			Subgroup: borderline	140–149	90–94
Stage 2	160–179	100–109	Grade 2	160–179	100–109
Stage 3	≥180	≥110	Grade 3	≥180	≥110
Isolated systolic hypertension	≥140	<90	Isolated systolic hypertension	≥140	<90
			Subgroup: borderline	140–149	<90

These guidelines are for people aged ≥18 years who are not taking antihypertensive drugs. When systolic and diastolic pressures fall into different categories, the higher category should apply. Blood pressure must be based on two or more readings on two or more visits.
*Phase V diastolic pressure (i.e. the disappearance of Korotkoff sounds).

report to avoid causing confusion; however, several subgroups were added to the WHO–ISH classification because their treatment recommendations differ from JNC recommendations in several respects. Both the JNC and WHO–ISH reports acknowledge the arbitrary nature of such classifications yet still place considerable emphasis on them. The other two sets of guideline (European and British) do not provide detailed classification based on blood pressure levels.

Discussion and recommendations

Given the continuous relationship between blood pressure and CVD risk, it is difficult to justify a detailed classification based on blood pressure levels except in the context of evidence of benefit from blood pressure-lowering therapy or in relation to the prognostic significance of different blood pressure levels. However, this is not the case with the classifications in the JNC and WHO–ISH reports. The continuous relationship between blood pressure and CVD risk is illustrated in *Fig. 3.1*, which shows the relative risks of stroke and of coronary heart disease (CHD) related to increasing diastolic blood pressure, from the combined results of a series of prospective observational studies.[6] Guidelines providing detailed classifications of blood pressure levels without a similar degree of detail in classifying other continuous CVD risk factors, such as age and lipid levels, are also likely to overemphasize the predictive value of

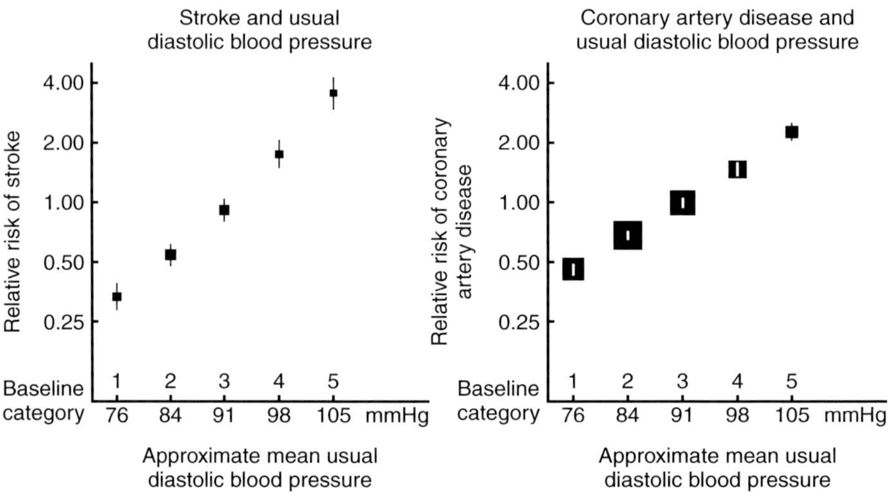

Figure 3.1

Relative risks of (a) stroke and (b) coronary artery disease in relation to diastolic blood pressure. (From the combined results of prospective observational studies.[6])

blood pressure in determining CVD risk. Moreover, as discussed below, blood pressure alone is a poor predictor of CVD risk in patients with mildly raised blood pressure.

Recommendation
It is recommended that classifications of blood pressure levels should be based only on the prognostic value of blood pressure levels or on levels at which treatment has been demonstrated to produce significant reductions in CVD risk. These issues are discussed below.

Blood pressure level treatment thresholds

The guidelines

Each of the four guidelines reviewed provides recommendations on drug treatment thresholds for specific patient groups, which are differentiated by blood pressure level and the presence or absence of other CVD risk factors. There are significant differences between the guidelines in treatment thresholds and timing of treatment (*Table 3.2*).

Thresholds irrespective of other risk factors
The JNC guidelines recommend initial lifestyle modification for those with blood pressure levels of 140–159 mmHg systolic and 90–99 mmHg diastolic unless target organ damage, diabetes mellitus, or clinical CVD is present. However, if blood pressure is sustained above 140/90 mmHg after 6 months in patients with one or more risk factors or after 12 months in patients with no other risk factors, then drug treatment is recommended. The WHO–ISH report recommends drug treatment for all patients with sustained blood pressure levels that are 10/5 mmHg higher than JNC thresholds at 150 mmHg systolic or 95 mmHg diastolic. As with JNC, the timing of treatment is dependent on other risk factors. The equivalent European and British recommendations for all patients irrespective of other risk factors advise drug treatment only when blood pressure is sustained at or above 160 mmHg systolic or 95 mmHg diastolic (European recommendations) and at or above 160 mmHg systolic or 100 mmHg diastolic (British recommendations).

Thresholds for patients with CVD risk factors
All four guidelines consider CVD risk factors in two general groups. The highest-risk group includes patients with clinical CHD or CVD, end-organ damage, or diabetes. Patients with dyslipidaemia or a family history of CHD and those who are older, male or smokers are considered separately.

For patients with clinical CVD, end-organ damage, or diabetes, JNC recommends drug treatment at blood pressure levels of ≥130 mmHg

Table 3.2 Recommended drug treatment thresholds in recent guidelines and thresholds recommended by the author

Patient group	Recommended drug treatment thresholds (mmHg)				
	JNC VI[9]	WHO–ISH[12]	European[11]	British[10]	Author
Irrespective of other CVD risk factors	≥140 systolic or ≥90 diastolic*	≥150 systolic or ≥95 diastolic	≥160 systolic or ≥95 diastolic	≥160 systolic or ≥100 diastolic	>about 170 systolic or >about 100 diastolic
With clinical CVD†	≥130 systolic or ≥85 diastolic	≥140 systolic or ≥90 diastolic	≥140 systolic or ≥90 diastolic	≥140 systolic or ≥85 diastolic	>about 150 systolic or >about 90 diastolic
End-organ damage‡	≥130 systolic or ≥85 diastolic	≥140 systolic or ≥90 diastolic	≥140 systolic or ≥90 diastolic	≥140 systolic or ≥90 diastolic	>about 150 systolic or >about 90 diastolic
With diabetes mellitus	≥130 systolic or ≥85 diastolic	≥130 systolic or ≥85 diastolic	≥140 systolic or ≥90 diastolic if estimated risk of CHD ≥20% in 10 years§	Type 1: ≥130 systolic or ≥80 diastolic Type II: ≥140 systolic if 10 yr risk of CHD ≥15% ≥140 systolic§	Type 1: >about 130 systolic or >about 80 diastolic Type II: >about 150 systolic or >about 90 diastolic if estimated 5 yr absolute CVD risk >about 10–15%§ and patient considers absolute CVD risk reduction from treatment to be worthwhile
With other CVD risk factors	≥140 systolic or ≥90 diastolic; risk factors only effect timing of treatment up to 1 year.	≥140 systolic or ≥90 diastolic, if one or more risk factors (assumes 10-year CVD risk ≥15%§)	≥140 systolic or ≥90 diastolic if estimated risk of CHD ≥20% in 10 years§	≥140 systolic or ≥90 diastolic, if estimated risk of CHD >15% in 10 years§ (=10 year CVD risk >20%)	>about 150 systolic or >about 90 diastolic if estimated 5 yr CVD risk >about 10–15%§ and patient considers absolute CVD risk reduction from treatment to be worthwhile

*Up to 12 months' lifestyle modification before treatment, depending on associated CVD risk factors.
†Clinical CVD includes angina, myocardial infarction, coronary revascularization, heart failure, stroke or transient ischemic attack, and peripheral arterial disease.
‡End-organ damage includes left ventricular hypertrophy, nephropathy, or retinopathy.
§Absolute risk of CVD estimated from tables provided with guidelines (based on Framingham Heart Study prognostic algorithms).
CVD, cardiovascular disease; CHD, coronary heart disease.

systolic or ≥85 mmHg diastolic. The WHO–ISH report recommends the same threshold for patients with diabetes or renal insufficiency but not for those with clinical CVD or end-organ damage. For these latter groups, the WHO–ISH reports recommends treatment at blood. pressure levels of ≥140 mmHg systolic or ≥90 mmHg diastolic. The European group recommends a treatment threshold of ≥140 mmHg systolic or 90 mmHg diastolic for patients with clinical CVD or end-organ damage and for the subgroup of diabetics who have an estimated 10-year risk of CHD ≥20%. Treatment is recommended for type 1 diabetics at blood pressure levels of ≥130 mmHg systolic or ≥80 mmHg diastolic in the British guidelines. For patients with clinical CHD and for those with type II diabetes who also have a risk of CHD ≥15% in 10 years, the British group recommend a blood pressure treatment threshold of ≥140 mmHg systolic or ≥85 mmHg diastolic.

For patients without clinical CVD, end-organ damage, or diabetes, the presence of other CVD risk factors influences only the timing of treatment in the JNC guidelines, and all patients with sustained blood pressure levels at or above 140/90 mmHg are recommended for drug treatment. The WHO–ISH report recommends the same 140/90 mmHg threshold if patients have at least one other CVD risk factor—these patients are assumed to have a 10-year risk of CVD risk of more than about 15%. The European and British groups recommend the 140/90 mmHg threshold if patients have a calculated 10-year risk of CHD risk ≥20% and ≥15%, respectively, based on risk charts provided with the guidelines.

Discussion and recommendations

The specific blood pressure level treatment thresholds recommended by the four guidelines are not well justified on trial evidence, although the British and European groups are the most explicit about the rationale for choosing cut-off levels. The general rationale given in all guidelines is that the higher the risk of CHD (or CVD), the lower the blood pressure treatment threshold should be.

Guideline thresholds irrespective of other risk factors
The major difference between treatment thresholds in the four guidelines is for patients irrespective of other risk factors. These vary from 140/90 mmHg to 160/100 mmHg. As illustrated in *Fig. 3.2*, which is based on a representative population sample aged 35–84 years from Auckland, New Zealand,[13] these different thresholds have a major impact on the numbers of patients who would be eligible for drug treatment. The JNC criteria define approximately 7% of the population aged 35–44 years as possibly eligible for drug treatment, rising to about 60% of the population aged 65–84 years. The equivalent percentages of eligible patients using WHO–ISH criteria are approximately 5% of those aged 35–44 years

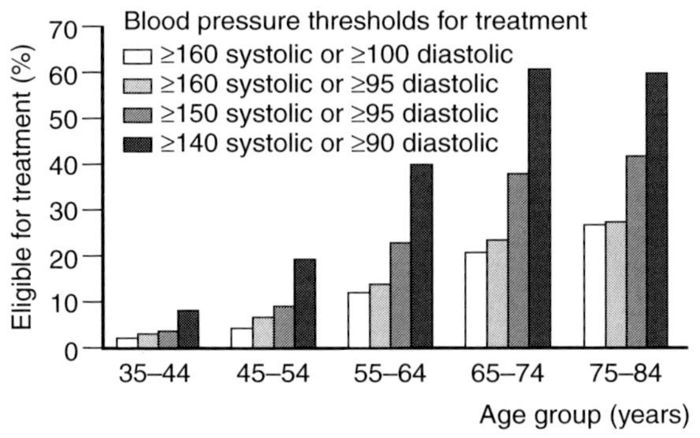

Figure 3.2

The effect of different blood pressure thresholds for treatment on the proportion of a population eligible for drug treatment. (Derived from a representative population sample.[13])

and 35–40% of those aged 65–84 years. If the European or British recommendations are followed, about 2% of those aged 35–44 years and about 20–25% of those aged 65–84 years would meet treatment criteria, regardless of other risk factors.

The implicit justification for these recommended blood pressure thresholds irrespective of other CVD risk factors is that the CVD risk in all such patients is too high to be left untreated. However. none of the guidelines appears to have quantified the magnitude of this risk, which probably accounts for the major differences between the recommendations. It would seem logical to choose a blood pressure threshold level for treatment, irrespective of other risk factors, at a point on the risk curve where the level of CVD risk associated with blood pressure is high whatever the associated risk factors. However, this level is above any of the thresholds recommended in the four guidelines and, based on the author's experience, also above levels that are likely to be acceptable to practitioners. A draft blood pressure management guideline was circulated by the author to a group of experts in the field in New Zealand, recommending a blood pressure level of 180 mmHg systolic or 105 mmHg diastolic as the treatment threshold irrespective of other risk factors. This level was consistently considered unacceptably high and consensus was reached at a level of 170 mmHg systolic and 100 mmHg diastolic (unpublished data).

Guideline thresholds for patients with other CVD risk factors

The recommended blood pressure thresholds for patients with symptomatic CVD, end-organ damage, or diabetes are more consistent between guidelines than for patients irrespective of other risk factors, but there remain significant differences. The JNC recommended cut-off of 130/85 mmHg for patients with CVD or end-organ damage and for all diabetic patients is only recommended by the WHO–ISH report for diabetics and for patients with renal insufficiency. The British guidelines recommend a similar threshold

Table 3.3 Approximate association between systolic and diastolic blood pressure by age in a representative population sample*

Systolic/diastolic blood pressure (mmHg) by age group	
35–54 years	55–74 years
165/100	185/100
145/90	165/90
130/80	145/80
110/70	130/70

*Blood pressure rounded to the nearest 5 mmHg.

only for type 1 diabetics, while the lowest European blood pressure threshold for any group is 140 mmHg systolic or 90 mmHg diastolic.

The most consistently recommended thresholds for patients with previous CVD are 140 mmHg systolic and 85–90 mmHg diastolic. These blood pressure thresholds are not directly supported by trials of blood pressure lowering since few trials have specifically examined antihypertensive treatment in this high-risk group. However, indirect support comes from trials that have used β-blockers and angiotensin converting enzyme (ACE) inhibitors in patients after myocardial infarction, although for reasons other than their blood pressure-lowering effects. Trials of long-term β-blockade in normotensive patients after myocardial infarction have demonstrated significant reductions in the risk of CHD.[14] ACE inhibitor treatment in normotensive patients with left ventricular failure, which is mainly secondary to myocardial infarction, have also been shown to reduce CHD event rates significantly.[15] Several trials of blood pressure lowering in hypertensive stroke survivors indicate a significant reduction in stroke risk, but trials in normotensive patients are inconclusive.[16]

The JNC and WHO–ISH groups appear to base their low blood pressure thresholds for all diabetic patients primarily on trials in normotensive type 1 diabetics. ACE inhibitors have been shown to slow the rate of decline in renal function in normotensive type 1 diabetics[17] and also to reduce progression of retinopathy in these patients.[18] Indirect evidence for the low threshold in diabetic patients comes from two recently published trials: the HOT trial,[19] which investigated three different blood pressure goals in hypertensive patients, including type II diabetics with raised blood pressure,[17] and the UKPDS trial,[20] which investigated two treatment goals in type II diabetics with treated or untreated hypertension. Although the recommendation for treating type 1 diabetics at thresholds of 130/80–85 mmHg is based on reasonable trial evidence, the same recommended threshold for type II diabetics is less defensible. Treatment thresholds were 100 mmHg diastolic in the HOT trial (mean entry levels of 170 mmHg systolic and 105 mmHg diastolic) whereas they were 160/90 mmHg (untreated) or 150/85 mmHg (treated) in UKPDS (mean entry levels of 160 mmHg systolic and 94 mmHg diastolic). Moreover, the mean blood pressure levels achieved through treatment were 144/85 mmHg, 141/83 mmHg and 140/81 mmHg in HOT and 154/87 mmHg and 144/82 mmHg in UKPDS.

The most consistent thresholds recommended in the guidelines for patients with other risk factors were also 140 mmHg systolic or 90 mmHg diastolic, although the definitions used for classifying other risk factors vary considerably (Table 3.4). As described in the next section a number of randomized trials demonstrating a significant treatment benefit have used a diastolic blood pressure cut-off of 90 mmHg and have given good justification for this diastolic threshold; however, the 140 mmHg systolic blood pressure threshold cannot be easily justified.

Associations between systolic and diastolic blood pressure levels

The most commonly recommended systolic/diastolic threshold combinations given in current guidelines (*Table 3.2*) are: 130/85, 140/90, 150/95, and 160/100 mmHg. However usual systolic/diastolic combinations in representative population samples (see Table 3.3) suggest that systolic pressures should be higher for the given diastolic pressures, particularly for people over 55 years, who represent the majority of hypertensive patients.

There is a strong correlation between systolic and diastolic blood pressure, and both measures have a similar association with CVD risk; therefore, it is appropriate to use systolic and diastolic thresholds that are consistent with each other. As illustrated in *Table 3.3*, a level of about 170 mmHg is a more appropriate systolic threshold level consistent with the diastolic threshold of about 100 mmHg; these levels are consistent with data from a range of studies.[21,22]

Table 3.4 lists the blood pressure level entry criteria plus the average entry and end blood pressure levels from the major randomized controlled trials of antihypertensive treatment.[23–34]

Although five of the 11 trials in *Table 3.4* had entry thresholds of ≥90 mmHg diastolic, the average diastolic entry level was 100 mmHg and the average systolic entry level was 171 mmHg. It is of note that the average end diastolic level in treated patients was 85 mmHg and the average end treated systolic level was 147 mmHg. Only one of the 11 trials had entry criteria with 150 mmHg systolic as the lower limit, and the mean entry systolic was 156 mmHg in this trial. There were four trials with a systolic entry threshold of ≥160 mmHg; the mean entry systolic was 178 mmHg in these trials and the mean end treated systolic was 149 mmHg. No trials had a mean entry systolic <150 mmHg.

In summary, a number of trials with entry thresholds of 90 mmHg

Table 3.4 Blood pressure level entry criteria, mean entry and end levels in placebo-controlled, randomized trials of antihypertensive drug treatment

Trial	Mean age; range (years)	Entry blood pressure criteria (systolic/diastolic) (mmHg)	Mean entry blood pressure (systolic/diastolic) (mmHg)	Mean end-of-trial blood pressure (treated) (systolic/diastolic) (mmHg)	Mean end-of-trial blood pressure (control) (systolic/diastolic) (mmHg)
VA II[25] (↓ stroke)	51; 24–75	—/90–114	164/104	135/86	169/106
HDFP stratum I[26] (↓ stroke and CHD)	51; 30–69	—/90–104	152/96	—/83	—/88
Oslo[27] (↓ stroke)	45; 40–49	150–179/<110	156/97	128/84	148/93
ANBPS[28] (↓ stroke)	50; 30–69	<200/95–109	157/100	—/88	—/94
MRC[29] (↓ stroke)	52; 35–64	<200/90–109	161/98	138/86	149/92
EWPHE[30] (↓ CHD)	72; 60–	160–239/90–119	183/101	149/85	172/94
HEP[31] (↓ stroke)	69; 60–79	170–280/105–120	196/99	162/77	180/88
SHEP[32] (↓ stroke and CHD)	72; 60–80	160–219/<90	170/77	144/68	155/71
STOP[33] (↓ stroke)	76; 70–84	180–230/90–120	195/102	166/85	193/95
MRC, older[34] (↓ stroke)	70; 65–74	160–209/<115	185/91	151/77	164/82
Syst-Eur[24] (↓ stroke)	70; 60–	160–219/<95	174/86	151/79	161/84

Only trials demonstrating significant reductions in CHD (↓ CHD) or stroke (↓ stroke) events rates or both (↓ stroke and CHD) included.
Data extracted from a comprehensive Swedish review (The Swedish Council on Technology Assessment in Health Care)[23] and from Staessen *et al.*[24]

diastolic have demonstrated significant reductions in CVD end-points, however no major trials have used systolic thresholds lower than about 150–160 mmHg. Moreover, it is unclear why all four guidelines examined present a systolic/diastolic combination threshold of 140/90 mmHg. As demonstrated in *Table 3.3*, the typical systolic blood pressure associated with a diastolic blood pressure of 90 mmHg is about 145 mmHg in people aged under 55 years and about 165 mmHg in the main group of hypertensive patients, who are over the age of 55 years.

Recommendation

Evidence from clinical trials assessing CVD end-points indicates that patients with systolic blood pressure above about 150 mmHg or diastolic blood pressure above about 90 mmHg will receive some benefit from blood pressure-lowering drugs. It is therefore recommended that patients with blood pressure levels above these levels should be offered drug treatment if the estimated magnitude of the absolute benefits of treatment (see below) is considered worthwhile by the patient. The trials do not help determine the threshold at which all patients should be recommended for drug treatment, irrespective of other CVD risk factors (i.e. irrespective of the estimated absolute risk and benefit of drug therapy). As illustrated in *Fig. 3.1*, cohort studies show a continuous relationship between blood pressure levels and relative CVD risk, with no obvious threshold. However when cohort studies present the relationship between blood pressure and absolute CVD risk, the risk slopes typically rise more markedly at blood pressure levels above 170/100 mmHg. Therefore a blood pressure level of about 170/100 mmHg is a reasonable threshold for recommending treatment for all patients, irrespective of estimated risk. In patients with blood pressure levels below about 150 mmHg systolic or 90 mmHg diastolic, a decision to offer drug treatment is an extrapolation from the trial evidence, with the possible exception of patients with type 1 diabetes mellitus, among whom thresholds of about 130 mmHg systolic or about 80–85 mmHg diastolic can be justified on trial evidence. Trials of blood pressure lowering in high-risk patients with blood pressure levels below about 150 mmHg systolic and 90 mmHg diastolic should be a high priority for research, given the significant potential for benefit in this group.

Timing of treatment

The guidelines

There are significant differences between guidelines regarding acceptable periods of monitoring and lifestyle modification before instituting treatment. In all guidelines, the timing of drug treatment is related to the level of blood pressure or the level of absolute CVD risk, or both, but none of the guidelines provides explicit justification for their recommendations.

Discussion and recommendations

It is inappropriate to specify a specific time period of observation and lifestyle management. Rather, patients and practitioners should be made aware that significant treatment effects are not apparent for at least 6–12 months and that the decision to start drug treatment should be based on the estimated probability of a CVD event without treatment over this period and their judgement of the likelihood that patients will make significant lifestyle changes. Although there is little trial evidence of the relative effectiveness of pharmacological versus non-pharmacological interventions in lowering CVD risk, there is good evidence that drug treatment lowers blood pressure more effectively than non-pharmacological methods.[35]

Recommendation
The key to the timing of drug treatment is to balance the likely risks and benefits of delaying treatment. Although the benefits are well documented and there appear to be no major risks associated with drug treatment, the decision to treat is usually a decision to treat for life. Clearly, the most desirable option is for patients to achieve a significant reduction in their blood pressure and other risk factors without drugs. In very high-risk patients, with predicted risk of major CVD events of 5–10% or more per year, a matter of a few weeks of lifestyle modification is reasonable before reassessing the patient for consideration of drug treatment. In patients with risks of, say, 2–5% per year, 3–6 months may be more appropriate before risk is reassessed. If the risk is lower than a few percent per year then a 12–24 month trial of lifestyle modification is worth considering before embarking on drug treatment.

Consideration of other CVD risk factors in treatment decisions

The guidelines

Each of the four guidelines explicitly considers other risk factors in their treatment recommendations (*Table 3.5*). The JNC guidelines provide the simplest classification based on three risk groups, but they are also the only guidelines that do not provide information on the magnitude of absolute risk or treatment benefit by risk group. All patients with clinical CVD, end-organ damage or diabetes are classified as high risk by JNC and recommended for immediate drug treatment at a threshold of 130 mmHg systolic or 85 mmHg diastolic. Patients with one other major risk factor are considered at medium risk and recommended for treatment at a threshold of 140 mmHg systolic or 90 mmHg diastolic after 6 months of lifestyle modification. The same threshold is recommended for patients with no major risk factors after 12 months of lifestyle modification.

The WHO–ISH guidelines provide the most complex categorization of risk that combines three grades of hypertension (see *Table 3.1*) and four categories of other risk factors:

(a) no other risk factors;
(b) one or two other risk factors;
(c) three or more risk factors, end-organ damage, or diabetes; and
(d) clinical CVD.

The combination of the blood pressure grades and other CVD risk factors categories classify patients into four risk groups, which are loosely assigned an absolute 10-year CVD risk. These risk estimates are stated to be based on calculations using CVD prediction algorithms from the Framingham Heart Study[36] applied to typical patients in each group. The risk groups are:

(a) low risk (assumed 10-year CVD risk <15%);
(b) medium risk (assumed 10-year CVD risk 15–20%);
(c) high risk (assumed 10-year CVD risk 20–30%); and
(d) very high risk (assumed 10-year CVD risk >30%).

The risk classification influences recommended timing of drug treatment and blood pressure thresholds for treatment, although the lowest blood pressure threshold (130 mmHg systolic or 85 mmHg diastolic) is reserved for diabetics, most of whom are assigned to the high-risk group (i.e. 20–30% 10-year CVD risk).

The European and British guidelines take a more specific quantitative approach to risk stratification. Patients with clinical CVD or end-organ damage are assigned to the highest risk group, as with JNC and WHO–ISH. However, all other patients, including diabetics, have their risk of coronary artery disease individually quantified using risk charts derived from the Framingham Heart Study. The charts are based on prognostic algorithms, which can estimate risk of CHD (or CVD) over a range of time periods using data on sex, age, diabetes status, smoking, blood lipid levels, and blood pressure levels.[36] Both the European and British charts use a 10-year risk period and calculate the risk of coronary artery disease rather than CVD risk, as used in the WHO–ISH classifications (CVD risk is typically about one-third higher than the risk of CHD). The European and British groups recommend shorter periods of lifestyle modification before drug treatment and lower blood pressure treatment

Table 3.5 CVD risk classification for patients with raised blood pressure used in guidelines and recommended by the author

JNC VI[9]	WHO–ISH[10]	European[11]	British[10]	The author
1. Risk Group C End-organ damage* or clinical CVD† or diabetes 2. Risk Group B At least one other risk factor 3. Risk Group A No other risk factors	1. Very high risk Grade 3 hypertension‡ and at least one other risk factor; or Grade 1 or 2 hypertension with clinical CVD (estimated 10-year CVD risk >30%) 2. High risk Grade 3 hypertension‡ or Grade 1 or 2 hypertension: with three or more risk factors or with diabetes or with end-organ damage (estimated 10-year CVD risk 20–30%) 3. Medium risk Grade 2 hypertension‡ or Grade 1 hypertension and one or two other risk factors (estimated 10-year CVD risk 15–20%) 4. Low risk Grade 1 hypertension with no risk factors (estimated 10-year CVD risk <15%)	1. Clinical CVD, end-organ damage, or 10-year CHD risk ≥20% (estimated using charts or computer algorithm derived from Framingham Heart Study data based on systolic blood pressure level, total cholesterol, age, sex, smoking, diabetes) 2. 10-year CHD risk <20% estimated as in 1. above	1. Clinical CVD, end-organ damage, or 10-year CHD risk ≥15% (estimated using charts or computer algorithm derived from Framingham Heart Study data based on systolic blood pressure level ratio of total - cholesterol to high density lipoprotein cholesterol, age, sex, smoking, diabetes) 2. 10-year CHD risk <15% estimated as in 1. above.	1. Clinical CVD, or end-organ damage (estimated 5-year CVD risk ≥15–20%) 2. Estimation of each patient's risk of CVD over 5 years using risk chart (see Fig. 3.4) 3. A 5-year CVD risk of about 10–15% is suggested as a level at which drug treatment should be considered (approximately equivalent to a 10-year CHD risk of 15–20%)

*End-organ damage includes left ventricular hypertrophy, nephropathy, or retinopathy.
†Clinical CVD includes angina, myocardial infarction, coronary revascularization, heart failure, stroke or transient ischemic attack, and peripheral arterial disease.
‡Grade of hypertension as defined in Table 3.1.
CVD, cardiovascular disease; CHD, coronary heart disease.

thresholds for higher-risk patients. The two guidelines differ slightly on the recommended level of absolute risk of CHD at which treatment should be initiated; however, both indicate that the levels are only guides. The British guidelines suggest a threshold of absolute CHD risk of about 15% over 10 years (equivalent to about a 20–25% CVD risk), whereas the Europeans recommend a threshold of 20% 10-year risk of coronary artery disease. However, the European guidelines recommend projecting the risk in patients aged less than 60 years to their risk at age 60 years, which reduces the difference between the risk thresholds of the two guidelines for younger patients.

Discussion and recommendations

There is currently a major paradigm shift under way in the management of hypertension (and dyslipidemia) with regard to the relevance of associated CVD risk factors. As illustrated in *Fig. 3.3*, which shows the 8-year risk of a CVD event in 40-year-old men from the Framingham Heart Study,[37] the prognostic influence of blood pressure is significantly influenced by the presence of other factors. For example, men with identical blood pressure levels but different risk profiles can have 15-fold differences in CVD risk. When age and sex are also considered, these differences are magnified even further, as shown in *Fig. 3.4*, which is a more comprehensive version of the Framingham Heart Study data in *Fig. 3.3*. *Figure 3.4*, which was developed in New Zealand[38–40] using the same Framingham data as was used in the British and European risk charts, estimates 5-year CVD risk and includes both men and women as well as younger and older people. *Figure 3.4* is very similar in appearance to the European guideline chart and very similar in content to the British chart. The differences between the charts are:

(a) the choice of a 5-year risk period and CVD risk in the New Zealand chart (see *Fig. 3.4*) rather than the 10-year period and risk of coronary artery disease in the European and British charts; and
(b) the inclusion of the ratio of total cholesterol to high-density lipoprotein (HDL) cholesterol in the New Zealand and British charts rather than total cholesterol alone as the lipid variable in the European chart.

Although the WHO–ISH guidelines do not include a risk chart, the CVD risk estimates given for their different categories are derived from the same Framingham data.

Trials of blood pressure-lowering drugs have shown remarkably similar relative CVD risk reductions across different risk categories,[2,41] with typical reductions in combined CVD mortality and morbidity of about one-quarter to one-third, particularly in those over 60 years of age, who represent the majority of treated hypertensives.[2] Therefore the absolute

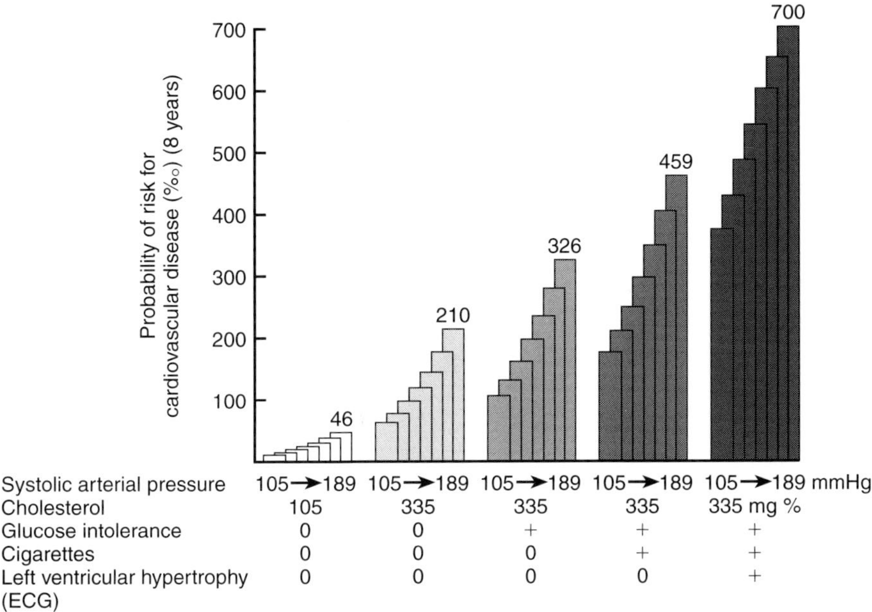

Systolic arterial pressure	105→189	105→189	105→189	105→189	105→189 mmHg
Cholesterol	105	335	335	335	335 mg %
Glucose intolerance	0	0	+	+	+
Cigarettes	0	0	0	+	+
Left ventricular hypertrophy (ECG)	0	0	0	0	+

Figure 3.3

Risk of cardiovascular disease according to the systolic blood pressure and associated risk factors in 40-year-old men. (Framingham Study: 18-year follow-up.[37])

benefits of antihypertensive drug treatment are directly related to a patient's pre-treatment risk of a CVD event. Despite similar relative risk reductions with treatment in younger and older patients, the absolute risk reductions in the higher-risk older patients were more than twice the absolute reductions in younger people.[2,41] Similar patterns have been observed in patient groups differentiated by other CVD risk factors.[2] One extreme example was observed in a comparison of stroke risk reduction in patients with and without a history of stroke. In both groups, a 38% relative reduction in stroke was observed; however, the absolute reduction in stroke risk was almost 10-fold greater in the group with a history of stroke, owing to their very high pre-treatment risk.[41]

Given the substantial differences in absolute benefits of blood pressure-lowering treatment related to pre-treatment CVD risk, it is clearly important to inform treatment decisions with information on a patient's pre-treatment risk. For some patients, such as those with previous symptomatic CVD or end-organ damage, their risk is known to be high; typically the 5-year risk of major CVD events in these patients is well over

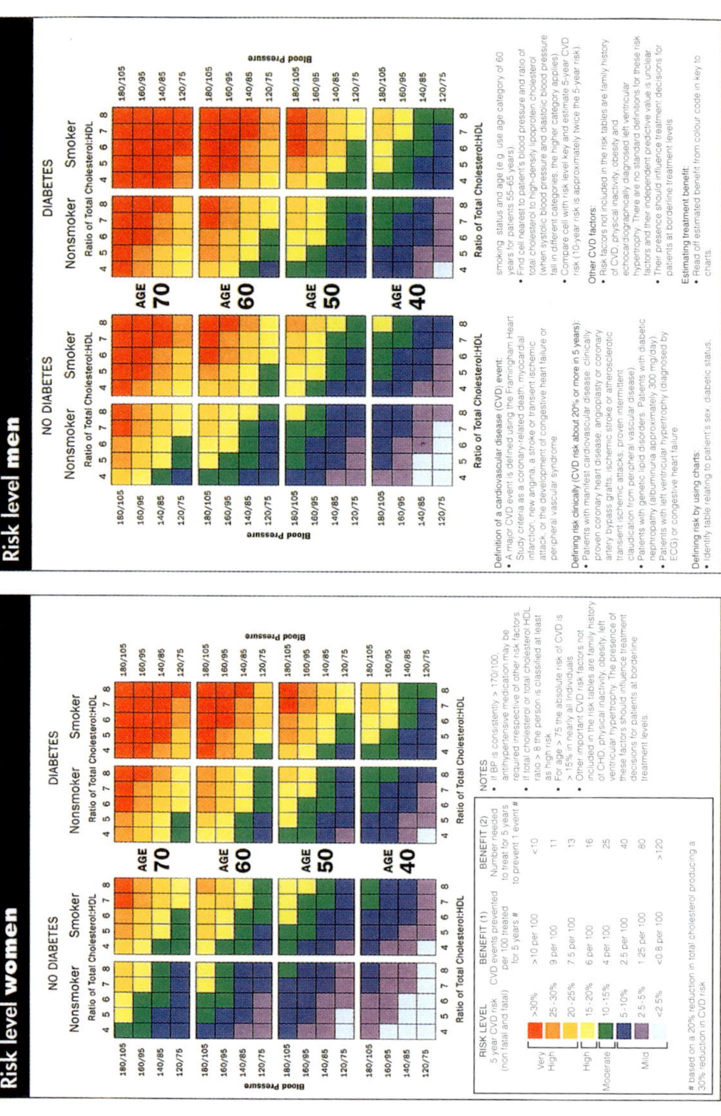

Figure 3.4

Cardiovascular disease: charts for quantifying risk and treatment benefits.[39,40]

20%. All guidelines classify these patients as being at high risk. However, for other patient groups, the guidelines vary markedly in their assessment of absolute risk and subsequent treatment recommendations.

Only the JNC recommendations rely on a qualitative risk classification alone. Although this has the advantage of simplicity, it can lead to gross misclassification of risk. For example, a 40-year-old non-smoking, non-diabetic male with a ratio of total cholesterol to HDL cholesterol of 4 and a blood pressure of about 160 mmHg systolic and 95 mmHg diastolic has a 5-year CVD risk of <2.5% (calculated from *Fig. 3.4*), but he is classified in the moderate risk group by JNC by virtue of his sex. In contrast, a 70-year-old non-diabetic, smoking male with the same blood pressure level but a ratio of total cholesterol to HDL cholesterol of 6 would have an estimated 5-year CVD risk more than 10-fold greater, at over 30% (calculated from *Fig. 3.4*) and is still classified as moderate risk by JNC. Moreover, all diabetic patients are classified along with patients with clinical CVD or end-organ damage in the highest JNC risk group despite estimated 5-year CVD risks of well under 5% in younger non-smoking diabetics (see *Fig. 3.4*).

The WHO–ISH guidelines loosely classified patients by absolute CVD risk; however, the attempts of these guidelines to simplify risk estimation have also resulted in significant misclassification of patient risk. All diabetics, for example, are classified in the high-risk group (i.e. 20–30% 10-year CVD risk) despite the low risk estimates in some diabetic patients described above. Moreover, the dichotomous classification of major CVD risk factors such as age (men >55 years and women >65 years), and dyslipidaemia (total cholesterol >6.5 mmol/l), can lead to major misclassification of risk.

In contrast, the approach taken by the European and British guidelines allows quantification of risk and, therefore, quantification of benefit of treatment in individual patients. The risk charts are relatively simple to use and, given that the decision to treat typically results in daily drug therapy for life, the few minutes required to quantify risk are easy to justify. The charts shown in *Fig. 3.4* go one step beyond the European and British charts by providing the estimated benefit of treatment as well as the pre-treatment risk. As discussed above, based on meta-analyses of treatment trials, it is assumed that the relative benefit of antihypertensive drug treatment is about one-third, whatever the pre-treatment risk. Although some have argued that the trials demonstrate a CVD risk reduction closer to one-quarter,[42] most trials have been of less than 5 years' duration and there has been considerable cross-over between treatment groups. Moreover, the estimates of benefit from meta-analyses are strongly influenced by older trials of younger low-risk people. These earlier trials, which used high doses of drugs, demonstrated smaller reductions in risk than in the more recent trials in older people, which have generally used lower doses of the same drugs. Therefore, a one-third relative reduction in combined fatal and non-fatal CVD is likely to be a reasonable estimate of the benefit of drug treatment. By combining the pre-treatment CVD risk based on the Framingham prognostic algorithms and the relative treatment benefit from meta-analyses of trials, the absolute benefit of treatment can be simply calculated by multiplying the pre-treatment risk by one-third. This benefit is expressed in *Fig. 3.4* as the events prevented per 100 people treated for 5 years and its reciprocal, which is the number of patients needing treatment for 5 years in order to prevent one event.

Whether a 5-year or a 10-year period of risk and benefit is used is of little consequence. This author favours a 5-year period since most treatment trials have been about 5 years' duration and a 5-year assessment may encourage more regular review of risk and management options. This author also favours assessing CVD risk rather than risk of CHD since treating hypertension reduces both and it is unnecessarily complicated to compute separate risks of CHD and stroke. Moreover, the predictive algorithms used in *Fig. 3.4* also take into account other major CVD events, including congestive heart failure and symptomatic peripheral vascular disease.

None of the quantitative risk charts takes account of the extra additional potential years of life gained when an event is prevented in a younger patient compared with those gained in an older patient, although the European chart does so indirectly by projecting the risk of CHD in younger patients to age 60 years. However the importance of the additional potential years of life gained in younger patients is likely to be small for several reasons. First, fatal events account for a much greater proportion of the events included in the charts among older patients than they do among younger patients. Secondly, although expectation of future life at 50 years of age may be about 30 years, expectation of future life at 70 years of age is about 15 years; this two-fold difference in years of life remaining is more than balanced by the 3–4-fold differences in 5-year CVD risk between 50-year-olds and 70-year-olds who have similar risk profiles. Nevertheless, the risk charts would be improved by taking potential life years gained by treatment into account.

Recommendation

Given the direct association between pre-treatment CVD risk and the absolute benefits of antihypertensive treatment, it is recommended that CVD risk should be estimated in all patients who are being considered for treatment (i.e. those with blood pressure levels above about 150 mmHg systolic or about 90 mmHg diastolic).

Patients with clinical CVD or documented end-organ damage can be assigned to the highest-risk group (i.e. estimated 5-year CVD risk more than about 20%) by signs alone. In these patients treatment is likely to reduce 5-year CVD risk by about one-third (i.e. about seven or more events prevented per 100 treated for 5 years, giving a number needed to be treated for 5 years to prevent one event of about 10–15 or fewer).

Patients with blood pressure levels consistently above about 170 mmHg systolic or 100 mmHg diastolic are also assumed to be at high risk due to their blood pressure levels alone and are generally recommended for treatment regardless of their quantified risk. Some of these patients are likely to have a modest risk, however few clinicians are willing to leave them untreated.

For all other patients, it is recommended that a CVD risk prediction chart (e.g. as illustrated in *Fig. 3.4* or in the European and British guidelines) should be used to estimate 5-year or 10-year CVD risk and the likely benefit of drug treatment. Patients should be advised that drug treatment has been shown to reduce CVD risk, and they should be informed of their estimated risk of an event without treatment and the estimated benefit of treatment. The decision to treat should be a shared one taken by the patient and practitioner. There is no obvious treatment threshold; however, as a guide, patients should be informed that most recommendations that have assessed absolute risk of CHD or CVD recommend drug treatment at a CVD risk of about 10% or more over 5 years; this is equivalent to a 10-year risk of CHD of about 15–20%. Approximately 25 patients with this level of risk will require treatment for about 5 years to prevent one CVD event.

Conclusions

Despite the wealth of randomized trial evidence examining the risks and benefits of drug treatment of raised blood pressure, there remain significant differences between treatment recommendations produced by various groups of experts. Many of the recommendations involve significant extrapolations from the trial evidence, and the differences between recommendations reflect the degree of extrapolation made rather than differences in the interpretation of the evidence. The potential implications of simply changing a recommended threshold blood pressure level for treatment by 5–10 mmHg are substantial in terms of the proportion of a population defined as eligible for treatment, and therefore the rationale for recommendations should be made explicit.

With the exception of type 1 diabetic patients, the blood pressure threshold above which there is reliable evidence of treatment benefit is about 150 mmHg systolic or about 90 mmHg diastolic. Given that a decision to initiate drug treatment is typically a decision to initiate daily, lifelong therapy, it is essential that patients with blood pressures above these thresholds should be made aware of the likely magnitude of treatment benefits and that the decision to treat with drugs is informed by this knowledge. There are now a wide range of CVD risk and benefit assessment tools available to help inform treatment decisions, and this author would argue that a clinician cannot provide high-quality management of hypertensive patients without a quantitative estimate of a patient's likely risk of a CVD event over the next 5–10 years and the likely benefit of drug treatment.

The benefits of lowering blood pressure in high risk patients with blood pressure levels below about 150/90 mmHg have not been adequately investigated and should be a high priority for future trials, given both the substantial potential benefits of treatment in such patients and the large size of the patient group.

References

1. Gueyffier F, Bulpitt C, Boissel JP *et al.* Antihypertensive drugs in very old people: a subgroup meta-analysis of randomised controlled trials. Lancet 1999; 353: 793–796.

2. Mulrow CD, Cornell JA, Herrera CR *et al.* Hypertension in the elderly. Implications and generalizability of randomised trials. JAMA 1994; 272: 1932–1938.

3. Gueyffier F, Froment A, Gouton M. New meta-analysis of treatment trials of hypertension: improving the estimate of therapeutic benefit. J Human Hyp 1996; 10: 1–8.

4. Beto JA, Bansal VK. Quality of life in treatment of hypertension: a meta-analysis of clinical trials. Am J Hyp 1992; 5: 125–133.

5. Croog SH, Levine S, Testa MA. The effects of antihypertensive therapy on quality of life. N Engl J Med 1986; 314: 1657–1664.

6. MacMahon S, Peto R, Cutler J *et al.* Blood pressure, stroke and coronary heart disease. Part 1, prolonged differences in blood pressure: prospective observational studies corrected for regression dilution bias. Lancet 1990; 335: 765–774.

7. Alderman MH. Blood pressure management: individualised treatment based on absolute risk and the potential for benefit. Ann Intern Med 1993; 119: 329–335.

8. Jackson R, Sackett D. Guidelines for managing raised blood pressure: evidence-based or evidence-burdened? BMJ 1996; 313: 64–65.

9. Joint National Committee. The sixth report of the Joint National Committee on prevention, detection, evaluation, and treatment of high blood pressure. Arch Intern Med 1997; 157: 2413– 2446.

10. Anonymous. Joint British recommendations on prevention of coronary heart disease in clinical practice. British Cardiac Society, British Hyperlipidaemia Association, British Hypertension Society, endorsed by the British Diabetic Association. Heart 1998; 80 (suppl 2): S1–S29.

11. Wood D, De Backer G, Faergeman O *et al.* Prevention of coronary heart disease in clinical practice: recommendations of the Second Joint Task Force of European and other Societies on Coronary Prevention. Atherosclerosis 1998; 140: 199–270.

12. Guidelines Subcommittee. 1999 World Health Organization–International Society of Hypertension Guidelines for the Management of Hypertension. Guidelines Sub-

committee. J Hypertens 1999; 17: 151–183.

13. Jackson R, Lay Yee R *et al.* Trends in coronary heart disease risk factors in Auckland between 1982 and 1994. N Z Med J 1995; 108: 451–454.

14. Freemantle N, Cleland J, Young P *et al.* Beta blockade after myocardial infarction: systematic review and meta regression analysis. BMJ 1999; 318: 1730–1737.

15. Lonn EM, Yusef S, Jha P *et al.* Emerging role of angiotensin-converting enzyme inhibitors in cardiac and vascular protection. Circulation 1994; 90: 2056–2069.

16. Rogers A, Neal B, MacMahon S. The effects of blood pressure lowering in individuals with cerebrovascular disease: an overview of randomised controlled trials. Neurol Rev Int 1997; 2: 12–15.

17. Lewis EJ, Hunsicker LG, Bain RP, Rohde RD. The effect of angiotensin converting enzyme inhibition on diabetic nephropathy: the Collaborative Study Group. N Engl J Med 1993; 329: 1456–1462.

18. Chaturvedi N, Sjolie AK, Stephenson JM *et al.* Effect of lisinopril on progression of retinopathy in normotensive people with type 1 diabetes. Lancet 1998; 351: 28–31.

19. Hansson L, Zanchetti A, Carruthers SG *et al.* Effects of intensive blood pressure lowering and low-dose aspirin in patients with hypertension: principal results of the Hypertension Optimal Treatment (HOT) randomised trial. Lancet 1998; 351: 1755–1762.

20. UK Prospective Diabetes Study Group. Tight blood pressure control and risk of macrovascular and microvascular complications in type 2 diabetes: UKPDS 38. BMJ 1998; 317: 703–713.

21. Hypertension Detection and Follow-up Program Cooperative Group. Five year findings of the Hypertension Detection and Follow-up Program. II. Mortality by race, sex and age. JAMA 1979; 242: 2572–2577.

22. Burt VL, Cutler JA, Higgins M. Trends in the prevalence, awareness, treatment, and control of hypertension in the adult US population: data from the health examination surveys, 1960 to 1991. Hypertension 1995; 26: 60–69.

23. The Swedish Council on Technology Assessment in Health Care. Moderately Elevated Blood Pressure. J Intern Med 1995; 238 (suppl 737): 135–225.

24. Staessen JA, Fagard R, Thijs L *et al.* Randomised double-blind comparison of placebo and active treatment for older patients with systolic hypertension. Lancet 1997; 350: 757–764.

25. Veterans Administration Cooperative Study Group on Antihypertensive Agents. Effects of treatment on morbidity in hypertension: II Results in patients with diastolic blood pressure averaging 90 through 114 mmHg. JAMA 1970; 213: 1143–1152.

26. Hypertension Detection and Follow-up Program Cooperative Group. Five year findings of the Hypertension Detection and Follow-up Program. 1. Reduction in mortality in persons with high blood pressure, including mild hypertension. JAMA 1979; 242: 2562–2571.

27. Helgeland A. The Oslo Study. Am J Med 1980; 69: 725–732.

28. A report by the Management Committee of the Australian Therapeutic Trial in Mild Hypertension. Untreated mild hypertension. Lancet 1982; 1: 185–191.

29. Medical Research Council Working Party. MRC Trial of treatment of mild hypertension: principal results. BMJ 1985; 291: 97–104.

30. Amery A, Birkenhager W, Brixko P *et al.* Mortality and morbidity results from the European Working Party on High Blood Pressure in the Elderly Trial. Lancet 1985; i: 1349–1354.

31. Coope J, Warrender TS. Randomised trial of treatment of hypertension in the elderly in primary care. BMJ 1986; 293: 1145–1151.

32. SHEP Cooperative Research Group. Prevention of stroke by antihypertensive drug treatment in older persons with isolated systolic hypertension. Final results of the Systolic Hypertension in the Elderly Program (SHEP). JAMA 1991; 265: 3255–3264.

33. Dahlof B, Lindholm LH, Hansson L *et al.* Morbidity and mortality in the Swedish Trial in Old Patients with Hypertension (STOP-Hypertension). Lancet 1991; 338: 1281–1285.

34. MRC Working Party. Medical Research Council trial of treatment of hypertension in older adults: principal results. BMJ 1992; 304: 405–412.

35. Ebrahim S, Davey Smith G. Lowering blood pressure: a systematic review of sustained effects of non-pharmacological interventions. J Public Health Med 1998; 20: 441–448.

36. Anderson KV, Odell PM, Wilson PWF, Kannel WB. Cardiovascular disease risk profiles. Am Heart J 1991; 121: 293–298.

37. Kannel WB. Some lessons in cardiovascular epidemiology from Framingham. Am J Cardiol 1976; 37: 269–282.

38. Jackson R, Barham P, Maling T *et al.* The management of raised blood pressure in New Zealand. BMJ 1993; 307: 107–110.

39. National Health Committee. Guidelines for the management of mildly raised blood pressure in New Zealand. Wellington, New Zealand: Ministry of Health, 1995.

40. Dyslipidaemia Advisory Group. 1996 National Heart Foundation clinical guidelines for the assessment and management of dyslipidaemia. N Z Med J 1996; 109: 224–232.

41. MacMahon S, Rogers A. The effects of antihypertensive treatment on vascular disease: reappraisal of the evidence in 1993. J Vasc Med Biol 1993; 4: 265–271.

42. Ramsay LE, Ul Haq I, Yeo W, Jackson PR. Interpretation of prospective trials in hypertension: do treatment guidelines accurately reflect current evidence? J Hypertens 1996; 14 (suppl 5): S187–S194.

4
The initial choice of antihypertensive drug

Henry R Black

Introduction

High blood pressure is the most common disease-specific reason for people in the USA to visit a physician. It is one of the most common medical problems throughout the world and its prevalence is increasing dramatically as the developing world reduces its death rate from diseases caused by infection and poor nutrition. If more people adopt a Western lifestyle, the prevalence is likely to rise even further. Recent estimates are that hypertension was the fourth leading cause of disability in the world in 1990, exceeded only by malnutrition, perinatal problems and infectious disease. By 2020, Lopez and Murray[1] have estimated that ischemic heart disease and stroke, both of which are consequences of high blood pressure and other cardiovascular risk factors, will be the most and the fourth most important health problems in the world. Soon, no society, whether acculturated or not, will be able to avoid the need to try to reduce the impact of hypertension. All nations will need to design and implement cost-effective case finding and treatment programs.

Because this condition is so common, all physicians and other healthcare providers will encounter hypertensive patients on an almost daily basis. Moreover, because its impact on the health of the public is so large, all providers should be familiar with the ways of evaluating and treating hypertensive patients.

This chapter reviews one approach to choosing initial therapy. Since nearly half of the patients we treat will not require any more treatment, this choice is perhaps the most important. It must be done expertly and with attention to many factors. When selecting initial treatment, and also subsequent treatment, one size does *not* fit all. With so many lifestyle modification and pharmacologic options available to the clinician, the likelihood of making the wrong choice is too high for the decision to be a careless one. Fortunately, the clinician who is familiar with a few simple principles is very likely to serve his or her patient well.

The approach discussed here is similar to the one that was recently recommended by The Sixth Joint National Committee on the Prevention, Detection, Evaluation and Treatment of High Blood Pressure (JNC VI).[2]

The recommendations in JNC VI revised earlier US guidelines for choosing initial and follow-up antihypertensive therapy and recommended a different treatment approach from the one that had been suggested in previous reports. JNC VI based its guidelines not only on the level of BP (which represents the relative risk imparted by elevations in blood pressure) but also on the presence or absence of other antecedents (risk factors) and comorbid conditions (which represent the absolute or attributable risk) imparted by the combination of an elevated blood pressure and these factors. This change is a result of a greater appreciation of the importance of absolute risk on the resultant benefit of treatment (i.e. the number of events that are prevented with effective therapy). *Those patients and populations at the highest absolute risk almost always benefit the most from effective treatment.*

In earlier guidelines, relative risk was the primary consideration, and possibly the only one, that was used for recommending when therapy should be started. Relative risk is the ratio of the risk of events or mortality, or both, when an individual or a population with higher blood pressures is compared to another individual or population with lower blood pressures. Relative risk progressively increases as both systolic blood pressure (SBP) and diastolic blood pressure (DBP) rise. Absolute risk estimates the risk from that elevated blood pressure reading in an individual (or a group of individuals) and takes into account the other conditions that affect risk. Although hypertension is the risk factor that contributes most to overall cardiovascular disease and especially to stroke, there are many other important risk factors for cardiovascular disease, which also determine the likelihood that cardiovascular disease or premature death will occur. A young person with stage 3 hypertension (SBP $\geq$180 mmHg and/or DBP $\geq$110 mmHg) who is free of other risk factors or comorbid conditions is likely to be at less risk of a cardiovascular event than an older patient with stage 1 hypertension (SBP 140–159 mmHg and/or DBP of 90–99 mmHg) who also has diabetes mellitus, an elevated cholesterol level and left ventricular hypertrophy.

A 'directed' history and physical examination and routine laboratory evaluation should be performed to assess the level of risk in every hypertensive patient. Completing this evaluation does not require any special expertise or any extensive or expensive testing. The evaluation is designed to discover the characteristics of each individual patient (i.e. other cardiovascular risk factors, comorbid conditions or socioeconomic factors) that would assist the clinician in assessing risk and might also alter the choice of initial therapy.

Selecting treatment

Although lifestyle modification has value for all hypertensive patients, most will need pharmacological treatment. For a more complete discussion of lifestyle modification, see Chapter 2. JNC VI suggests that patients with stage 2 or 3 hypertension (SBP ≥160 mmHg or DBP ≥100 mmHg) and those in risk group C (those with diabetes mellitus and those with clinical cardiovascular disease) should in fact receive drug therapy once their hypertension has been diagnosed and confirmed. Furthermore, the length of time that the clinician should rely on lifestyle modifications before starting drug therapy has been clarified in JNC VI and is based on risk estimates, not just on the level of blood pressure (*Table 4.1*). Those with stage 1 hypertension (SBP 140–159 mmHg and/or DBP 90–99 mmHg) who have no other risk factors or end-organ damage (so-called risk group A) can be treated only with lifestyle modification for up to 1 year, even if goal blood pressure is not reached (see page 47), before drug therapy is considered to be necessary. While on the other hand, patients with stage 1 hypertension who are in risk group B (other risk factors but no end-organ damage or diabetes mellitus) should receive pharmacological therapy after only a 6-month trial of lifestyle modification, unless goal blood pressure is achieved without drugs. Since male sex and age over 60 years are considered risk factors, only women who are under 60 years of age are in group A. Those in risk group C (end-organ damage, clinical cardiovascular disease and diabetes mellitus) should be treated with pharmacological agents *and* lifestyle modification even if they have high normal blood pressure levels (SBP 130–139 mmHg and/or DBP 85–89 mmHg).

JNC VI recommended weight loss for obese hypertensive patients, modification of dietary sodium intake to ≤100 mmol/day, and modification of alcohol intake to no more than two drinks per day. It also recommended increased physical activity for all patients with hypertension who had no specific reason why such a recommendation was not applicable or safe. Yet for many of our patients these suggestions are either not practicable or are already being done. For such patients, drug therapy may be indicated even sooner in group A and group B hypertensive patients.

Pharmacological therapy

Basic principles

The choice of the drug with which to begin therapy is probably the most important decision the clinician must make when treating hypertensive patients. Approximately half of the patients we treat will respond to our first choice and can tolerate most of our rational options. If we choose wisely, our first choice will be successful in getting blood pressure to goal (see page 73), and that will be the drug our patient remains on for what is usually an indefinite period of therapy.

Table 4.1 Risk stratification and treatment of hypertension (modified from JNC VI[2])

Blood pressure stage (mmHg)	Risk group A (No risk factors, no end-organ damage, no clinical cardiovascular disease)	Risk group B (At least one risk factor not including diabetes mellitus, no end-organ damage, no clinical cardiovascular disease)	Risk group C (End-organ damage and/or diabetes mellitus, with or without other risk factors)
High normal (130–139/85–89)	Lifestyle modification	Lifestyle modification	Drug therapy
Stage 1 (140–159/90–99)	Lifestyle modification (for up to 12 months)	Lifestyle modification (for up to 6 months)	Drug therapy
Stages 2 and 3 (>160/>100)	Drug therapy	Drug therapy	Drug therapy

Classification of antihypertensive agents

Antihypertensive agents are classified in a number of ways. Some are effective parentally and are indicated only for a hypertensive crisis. Those discussed in this chapter are the ones that work orally and are used for the long-term management of high blood pressure. Antihypertensive agents are then further classified by their pharmacological class and their alleged primary mechanism of action (*Table 4.2*). Fortunately, there are more than 80 effective antihypertensive drugs and 40 fixed-dose combinations from which to choose. All of these agents lower blood pressure and, in appropriate doses, do so to essentially the same degree.

Surrogate versus clinical end-points

We are now no longer willing simply to look at the degree of blood pressure reduction when making our choice of antihypertensive therapy. Blood pressure reduction is a so-called surrogate or intermediate end-point. Since the reason that we treat hypertension is to reduce the morbidity and mortality associated with an elevated blood pressure and not to just lower blood pressure, we now expect proof that the drugs we choose favorably affect morbidity and mortality. Such data is only available from large and well-done clinical trials that evaluate the ability of a drug to reduce hypertension-related cardiovascular events as well as or better than another drug that we might choose.

Before 1997, only diuretics and β-blockers had been shown to reduce the morbidity and mortality in clinical trials in hypertension. Dihydropyridine calcium antagonists were added to the list after the Syst-EUR trial[3] was completed (see Chapter 5). This trial used nitrendipine, followed by

Table 4.2 Classification of oral antihypertensive drugs

Adrenergic inhibitors
   Peripheral agents
   Central α-agonists
   α-Blockers
   β-Blockers
   α–β-Blockers
Angiotensin converting enzyme inhibitors
Angiotensin II receptor blockers
Calcium antagonists
   Non-dihydropyridine calcium antagonists
   Dihydropyridine calcium antagonists
Direct vasodilators
Diuretics

enalapril and hydrochlorothiazide if needed to get blood pressure to goal.

Numerous studies have shown the value of angiotensin converting enzyme (ACE) inhibitors in saving lives of patients with heart failure, after a myocardial infarction and in those who have type 1 diabetes mellitus with nephropathy and proteinuria. Although many of the subjects in these trials were hypertensive, they were enrolled in the studies because they had these other conditions. It was only in 1999, when the Captopril Prevention Program (CAPPP) was published that benefit of this class of agents on morbidity and mortality in hypertensives was shown.[4] CAPPP showed that a regimen starting with captopril achieved the same benefit in reducing morbidity and mortality as one that began either diuretics or β-blockers (so-called conventional therapy). Interestingly, the group that was randomized to conventional therapy had statistically significantly fewer strokes and the group given the ACE inhibitors had a lower incidence of new diabetes mellitus and better outcomes in those with known type 2 diabetes mellitus.

In the next few years, approximately 30 more events trials will be completed.[5] When some or all of these trials are completed, we should know with some degree of certainty whether lowering blood pressure is all that matters or whether we should select particular classes of drugs because they prevent hypertension-related events more effectively. The largest of these trials, with 42,000 subjects, the Antihypertensive and Lipid Lowering Trial to Prevent Heart Attack (ALLHAT) is due to be completed in 2003.[6] ALLHAT will compare diuretics to dihydropyridone calcium antagonists, ACE inhibitors and α-blockers using ischemic heart disease as the primary end-point. The Controlled ONset Verapamil Investigation of Cardiovascular Endpoints (CONVINCE) is comparing a non-dihydropyridine calcium antagonist (verapamil) in 16,600 older hypertensives and should also be finished in 2003.[7] Trials of angiotensin II receptor blockers are also due to be finished by then.[5]

Individualizing therapy

In view of the many effective options available, we must pay very close attention to each patient's needs and plan his or her regimen accordingly. We must treat each patient as an individual, not as a member of a 'population' and so the drug that we choose must be compatible with that individual patient's lifestyle and job requirements. Whatever we select it must be affordable. No amount of therapeutic wisdom will be effective if our patient does not have the funds to purchase our choice.

Goal of therapy

We must strive to reduce SBP to below 140 mmHg *and* to reduce DBP to below 90 mmHg, the goal currently articulated by JNC VI and the more recent World Health Organization–International Society of Hypertension guidelines.[8] In diabetics, the recommended goal was lower (SBP < 130 mmHg and DBP < 85 mmHg). This was suggested by JNC VI before the publication of the Hypertension Optimal Treatment (HOT) study[9] and the United Kingdom Diabetes Prevention Study (UKDPS).[10] JNC VI recommended these more stringent goals for those with diabetes mellitus not because of 'evidence' from clinical trials but rather from the appreciation of the higher absolute risk that diabetics have and the expectation that lowering blood pressure further than 140/90 mmHg would be of particular benefit for this high-risk group. HOT and UKPDS provided the solid evidence that was needed to support this recommendation. In patients with renal disease and at least 1 g of proteinuria per day, JNC VI recommended an even lower goal (SBP < 125 mmHg and DBP < 75 mmHg).

While the benefits of this level of aggressive therapy has still not been proved conclusively, clinical trial results that are currently available do suggest that substantially more events would be prevented with these treatment goals than with higher levels, with little if any harm to the patient. An analysis by Elliott and colleagues[11] suggests that such an approach would actually save money, even though more drugs would be needed. The additional cost of drugs and follow-up visits is more than balanced by the presumed reduction in cardiovascular and renal events. The African American Study of Kidney Disease (AASK) is directly addressing the issue of blood pressure goal in those with renal impairment. This trial too will be completed within the next few years.

Factors in the choice of agents for antihypertensive therapy

There are eight factors that should always be considered when initial therapy is chosen and drugs are added (if additional agents are needed to reduce blood pressure to goal), and these are listed in *Table 4.3*.

Table 4.3 Factors in the choice of agents for antihypertensive therapy

Efficacy
Safety
Comorbidity and other risk factors
Special populations
Dosage schedule
Drug interactions
Cost
Mechanisms of action of the drug and pathophysiology of the patient's
   hypertension

Efficacy

JNC VI made the appropriate distinction between surrogate and clinical end-points in the selection of treatment. Clinical end-points are the events that we are trying to prevent when we treat hypertension. Surrogate (or intermediate) end-points are factors that may contribute to clinical end-points and that can be favorably or unfavorably affected by treatment. To date, four classes of drugs (thiazide diuretics, β-blockers, dihydropyridine calcium antagonists and ACE inhibitors) have been shown to reduce clinical end-points when used as the initial therapy for hypertension in appropriately designed and implemented clinical trials. Other agents such as peripheral sympatholytics (reserpine and guanethidine), centrally acting α_2-agonists (α-methyldopa) and vasodilators (hydralazine), have also been used in clinical trials as the second, third or even fourth agent to be added to get blood pressure under control. None is an option for initial therapy, either because they are relatively poorly tolerated compared with the agents that are recommended as initial therapy or because they need to be taken together with diuretics in order to lower blood pressure effectively in the long term. Other agents, such as α-blockers, α–β-blockers and angiotensin II receptor blockers, are effective as monotherapy and are well tolerated, but these drug classes have not, as yet, been shown to reduce clinical end-points.

JNC VI has also recognized two other factors that may alter the correct choice for initial treatment in an individual hypertensive patient:

(a) data from events trials that were conducted in subjects with other conditions (e.g. type 1 diabetes mellitus, acute myocardial infarction, heart failure) but in which many subjects with hypertension were enrolled—these were the basis for the JNC VI designation of a 'compelling' indication (*Table 4.4*);
(b) the fact that individual patients may have certain comorbid conditions for which a specific agent might be appropriate, although no trial has yet been completed in which that agent has been compared to drugs for which clinical trial data is currently available—this was the basis of the JNC VI recommendation for a drug to be indicated or contraindicated as a specific indication even though randomized clinical trials might not yet be available to support the decision (see *Table 4.4*).

This second approach was also used by The British Hypertension Society.[12] In their guidelines similar language was used, but they considered the presence of some of these comorbid conditions to be a compelling reason to choose a particular class of drugs even though a trial had not been completed proving the value of those agents in patients with these conditions.

Table 4.4 Considerations in individualizing antihypertensive drug therapy (modified from JNC VI[2])

Indication	Drug therapy
Compelling indications unless contraindicated	
Diabetes mellitus (type 1) with proteinuria	ACE inhibitors
Heart failure (systolic)	ACE inhibitors, diuretics, β-Blockers, aldosterone receptor blockers
Isolated systolic hypertension (older patients)	Diuretics (preferred), calcium antagonists (long-acting dihydropyridine)
Myocardial infarction	β-Blockers (non-ISA), ACE inhibitors (in cases of systolic dysfunction)
May have favorable effects on comorbid conditions	
Angina	β-Blockers, calcium antagonists
Atrial tachycardia and fibrillation	β-Blockers, CA (non-dihydropyridine)
Cyclosporine-induced hypertension (caution with the dose of cyclosporine)	Calcium antagonists
Diabetes mellitus (types 1 and 2) with proteinuria	ACE inhibitors (preferred), calcium antagonists
Diabetes mellitus (type 2)	Low-dose diuretics
Dyslipidemia	α-Blockers
Essential tremor	β-Blockers (non-cardioselective)
Heart failure (systolic)	Losartan potassium, β-blockers
Hyperthyroidism	β-Blockers
Migraine	β-Blockers (non-cardioselective), calcium antagonists (non-dihydropyridine)
Myocardial infarction	Diltiazem hydrochloride, verapamil hydrochloride
Osteoporosis	Thiazides
Preoperative hypertension	β-Blockers
Prostatism (benign prostatic hyperplasia)	α-Blockers
Renal insufficiency (caution in renovascular hypertension and creatinine > 3 mg/dl)	ACE inhibitors
May have unfavorable effects on comorbid conditions	
Bronchospastic disease	β-Blockers
Depression	β-Blockers, central α-agonists, reserpine
Diabetes mellitus (types 1 and 2)	β-Blockers, high-dose diuretics
Dyslipidemia	β-Blockers (non-ISA), diuretics (high-dose)
Gout	Diuretics
Second- or third-degree heart block	β-Blockers, calcium antagonists (non-dihydropyridine)
Heart failure	Calcium antagonists (except amlodipine besylate, felodipine)
Liver disease	Labetalol hydrochloride, methyldopa
Peripheral vascular disease	β-Blockers
Pregnancy	ACE inhibitors, angiotensin II receptor blockers
Renal insufficiency	Potassium-sparing agents
Renovascular disease	ACE inhibitors, angiotensin II receptor blockers

ACE, angiotensin converting enzyme; ISA, intrinsic sympathomimetic activity.

Adverse reactions and side effects

There are two primary types of adverse reactions and side effects that may occur with antihypertensive therapy: clinical and biochemical (*Table 4.5*). Clinical side effects are directly evident to the patient and are perceived by the patient or the clinician to be related to the drug. The appearance of these adverse reactions require that the drug be stopped, the dose be reduced or the patient be willing to remain on therapy until he or she becomes able to tolerate the side effect or it disappears. The drugs recommended for initial therapy generally cause fewer clinical side effects than other drugs at the doses that lower blood pressure.

Recently, a series of low-dose fixed-dose combinations have been introduced that have fewer clinical side effects than some of the components have when used as monotherapy. The best example is the combination of a dihydropyridine calcium antagonist with an ACE inhibitor. All of these fixed-dose combinations have a significantly lower incidence of edema than that seen when the dihydropropyridine calcium antagonist is given alone. The incidence of cough, however, is not lessened when these drugs are combined.

Biochemical side effects may lead to clinically evident adverse reactions (e.g. hypokalemia from thiazide diuretics causing muscle weakness, palpitations, nocturia or polyuria), but usually the biochemical problems that occur with antihypertensive agents are more troublesome to the provider than they are to the patient.

The importance of biochemical side effects is usually not that they result in clinically evident problems but the danger that these drug-related permutations of lipids, glucose or insulin may aggravate other risk factors and accelerate the clinical impact of dyslipidemias, glucose intolerance or insulin resistance. Whether the minor and often short-term effects on total serum cholesterol, high-density lipoprotein (HDL) cholesterol or triglycerides that result from therapy with thiazides or β-blockers are responsible for an increase in ischaemic heart disease remains to be proved.[13] At the doses that are now recommended, these changes and the electrolyte disturbances noted with thiazides are modest, although it is still possible that, at high doses, thiazides could reduce serum potassium sufficiently to increase the rate of sudden cardiac death. Whether the increases in insulin resistance that are seen with thiazide diuretics and β-blockers or the hypokalemia that is seen with thiazide diuretics have precipitated diabetes mellitus sooner or in patients who would not otherwise have become diabetic also remains to be proved. Although it is not certain that these metabolic adverse reactions are clinically relevant, it may be prudent to select another option for patients with diabetes mellitus or a dyslipidemia, so long as blood pressure is successfully reduced to goal. Certain types of dual therapy may also ameliorate biochemical adverse reactions (ACE inhibitors (and angiotensin receptor blockers)

Table 4.5 Selected important adverse reactions to antihypertensive agents

Drug	Adverse effects	
	Clinical	Biochemical
Diuretics		
Thiazides	Weakness	Hypokalemia
	Sexual dysfunction	Hyponatremia
	Diabetes mellitus	Hypomagnesemia
	Gout	Hyperglycemia
		Hypertriglyceridemia
		Hypercholesterolemia
		Hyperuricemia
		Hypercalcemia
		Reduction HDL cholesterol
Loop-active agents	Volume depletion	Same as thiazides except not hypercalcemia
Potassium-sparing agents	Gynecomastia and breast tenderness	Hyperkalemia (all)
	Sexual dysfunction	
	Menstrual irregularities (spironolactone only)	
Sympatholytics		
β-Blockers	Fatigue	Hypertriglyceridemia
	Bronchospasm	Reduction in HDL cholesterol
	Intermittent claudication	Hyperglycemia
	Bradycardia and heart block	
	Systolic dysfunction	
	Sleep disturbances	
	Diabetes mellitus	
Peripheral α_1-adrenoreceptor	Syncope	
	Orthostatic hypotension	
	Headache	
	Syncope	
	Orthostatic hypotension	
Central α_2-agonists	Headache	
	Sedation	
	Dry mouth	
	Orthostatic hypotension	
	Fatigue	
	Rebound hypertension	
	Liver toxicity (methyldopa)	
	Hemolytic anemia (methyldopa)	
Peripherally acting sympatholytics	Rash (clonidine patch)	
	Orthostatic hypotension	
	Retrograde ejaculation (guanethidine)	
	Lethargy	
	Depression (reserpine)	
	Dizziness (reserpine)	
	Dyspepsia	
Angiotensin-converting enzyme inhibitors	Cough	Hyperkalemia
	Angioedema	
	Renal failure	
Angiotensin receptor blockers	Renal failure	Hyperkalemia
Calcium antagonists		
Non-dihydropyridine calcium antagonists	Bradycardia	
	Heart block	
	Constipation (verapamil)	
	Headache (diltiazem)	
Dihydropyridine calcium antagonists	Headache	
	Dizziness	
	Edema	
	Palpitations	
Direct vasodilators	Palpitations	
	Edema	
	Headache	
	Hirsutism (minoxidil)	

HDL, high density lipoprotein.

and thiazides, when given together, produce few if any of the metabolic abnormalities associated with thiazides alone. Several fixed-dose combinations or these classes of drugs are available and may be appropriate as initial therapy.

The incidence of clinical side effects tends to rise with increasing doses with all classes of drugs, with the exception of ACE inhibitors and angiotensin receptor blockers. Patients who develop an adverse reaction on a high dose of a drug or on a dose that they previously tolerated do not necessarily need to have that drug discontinued. Rather, the dose can be lowered and another antihypertensive added to reduce blood pressure to goal. The primary problems with ACE inhibitors are cough and angioedema, both of which tend to be idiosyncratic and occur with all representatives of that class of agents. Reducing the dose or changing to a different ACE inhibitor is rarely helpful. ACE inhibitors should be increased to the maximum recommended dose before therapy is abandoned or another agent is added. Angiotensin II receptor blockers as a class appear to be the best tolerated of all currently available antihypertensive agents. Although some experts feel that they should be reserved for initial therapy only in patients who developed a cough with ACE inhibitors, they are also an excellent option for patients who have no complaints when treatment is being started and for patients in whom a drug that primarily blocks the renin–angiotensin–aldosterone system (see Chapter 7) appears to be a good option.

Comorbidity and other risk factors

The presence of other risk factors or active clinical problems may alter the initial and subsequent choice of antihypertensive therapy in an individual patient. The appreciation that the drugs that we prescribe to reduce blood pressure can either improve or adversely effect other clinical conditions is the basis for the JNC VI recommendation that, although diuretics and β-blockers should be used when a patient has 'uncomplicated' hypertension, the presence of these comorbid conditions may and should alter the choice of initial therapy, even though there is no trial to support the recommendation (see *Table 4.4*).

It is highly unlikely, for example, that we will ever have a study that shows the benefit of peripheral α-blockers compared with other antihypertensive agents in men with prostatic hypertrophy, but any prudent clinician would consider it wise to treat both conditions with a single agent since it is possible to do so. There are many other examples of how this principle should be applied, as discussed below.

Dyslipidemias

Hypertensive patients who have lipid abnormalities (which may be present in as many as 50% of those treated for hypertension) probably should not be treated with drugs that worsen their particular dyslipidemia. Although it has not as yet been proved that the changes in serum lipids caused by certain classes of antihypertensive agents are harmful, it is certainly reasonable to choose an equally effective drug that is lipid-neutral or to choose one that may even improve the lipid profile. In large doses (> 25 mg/day), thiazide diuretics and related compounds, such as chlorthalidone, raise total serum cholesterol and low-density lipoprotein (LDL) cholesterol by 5–10%, at least transiently, and may lower HDL cholesterol by 2–4%.[13] Serum triglyceride is increased by 15–30%. With the doses that are currently recommended (using up to but no more than 25 mg of hydrochlorothiazide), there is little if any alterations in these parameters. β-Blockers that do not have intrinsic sympathomimetic activity lower HDL cholesterol even more (10%) and also raise triglycerides (by approximately 20%) without affecting total cholesterol or LDL cholesterol. β-Blockers that do have intrinsic sympathomimetic activity and α–β-blockers are lipid-neutral.

On the other hand, one could choose to initiate therapy with a peripheral α-blocker in patients who have dyslipidemias. These drugs reduce total cholesterol and LDL cholesterol by approximately 8–10%, triglycerides by 15% and HDL cholesterol by 10–15%. Although these alterations are modest, the overall cardiovascular risk of a hypertensive patient whose lipids are changed in this fashion is clearly lessened. ACE inhibitors do not affect serum lipids, and in some studies benefits similar to those seen with α-blockers have been observed. Angiotensin receptor blockers and calcium antagonists are lipid-neutral. ALLHAT will help to define whether drugs that affect the lipid profile, whether in a seemingly beneficial or adverse direction, truly affect the occurrence of ischemic heart disease or other atherosclerotic complications.[6]

Other sympatholytics do not affect the lipid profile, and direct vasodilators (e.g. hydralazine) raise HDL cholesterol and lower total cholesterol, cholesterol and triglycerides, even when used in combination with thiazide diuretics.

Glucose and insulin

Antihypertensive drugs may affect glucose metabolism and may worsen or improve insulin sensitivity. The magnitude and direction of the drug-induced changes seen in glucose and insulin are very similar to that which occurs with lipids. Peripheral α-blockers and some ACE inhibitors (captopril, enalapril, and perindopril) may improve insulin sensitivity. Not only do some ACE inhibitors improve insulin sensitivity, most have also been shown to reduce urinary protein excretion, which may contribute to the renal benefit seen in patients with diabetes mellitus. Both thiazides and β-blockers worsen insulin sensitivity and may occasionally precipitate glucose intolerance, but rarely do these drugs cause clinical diabetes mellitus. In spite of these metabolic changes, in the Systolic

Hypertension in the Elderly Program (SHEP),[14] treatment with low-dose chlorthalidone (plus atenolol or reserpine in some volunteers) reduced clinical events in the diabetic subgroup, even more so than occurred in the non-diabetics.[14]

There are very few data on other classes of antihypertensive agents, although some preliminary studies with angiotensin II receptor blockers (particularly candasartan and irbesartan) are promising. JNC VI recommended that only hypertensive patients with type 1 diabetes mellitus should be given ACE inhibitors (a compelling indication) because the only randomized clinical trial that has clearly demonstrated the utility of ACE inhibitors in reducing clinical events was done in a group of type 1 diabetic patients with hypertension.[15] Although there are no large, long-term events trials yet completed that have proved any special value of ACE inhibitors in patients with type 2 diabetes mellitus, many feel that the benefit shown for type 1 diabetic patients can also be assumed to occur for type 2 diabetic patients. Others argue that if blood pressure control is achieved, it does not matter what drug or drugs are used. In UKPDS, the group that received the ACE inhibitor captopril did no better than the group that received atenolol, which lends some support to the argument that it is blood pressure control and how it is accomplished that is the key factor in type 2 diabetic patients.[10]

Although some experts have raised concerns about the safety of dihydropiridine calcium antagonists in type 2 diabetic patients, the Syst-EUR study, in which these drugs were the initial therapy, recently demonstrated that the benefit accrued was greater in the diabetic patients than it was in other patients.[16] Just as with SHEP, the results of a properly done clinical trial refuted contentions based on notions from smaller human studies and animal experiments. Non-dihydropiridine calcium antagonists alone and in combination with ACE inhibitors may also lower urinary protein and thus be particularly useful in diabetic patients with nephropathy. At this time, it would appear that no drugs are contraindicated in hypertensive patients with diabetes mellitus and that what is most important is reducing blood pressure to goal (<130/85 mmHg, or < 125/75 mmHg if nephropathy and heavy proteinuria are present).

Left ventricular hypertrophy

Left ventricular hypertrophy is a common consequence of hypertension and a robust independent risk factor for cardiovascular disease and premature mortality. It is especially common in the elderly, particularly in elderly women, and it is often associated with diastolic dysfunction. It appears that all antihypertensive agents that are recommended for initial therapy reduce left ventricular mass. Data from meta-analyses have suggested that agents that block the renin–angiotensin–aldosterone system reduce left ventricular mass better than other antihypertensive agents.[17,18] However, neither the Treatment Of Mild Hypertension Study (TOMHS)[19] nor the most recent Veterans Administration Trial of Monotherapy,[20] which compared agents from a number of drug classes used as monotherapy, supported this contention. In these trials, drugs were assigned in a randomized fashion and the comparison was prospectively designed. In both trials, all classes of commonly used antihypertensive agents successfully reduced left ventricular mass; surprisingly, thiazide diuretics were the most successful.

Systolic and diastolic dysfunction and heart failure

In patients with heart failure caused by systolic dysfunction, ACE inhibitors, diuretics (loop-active agents and aldosterone receptor blockers such as aldactone) and possibly angiotensin II receptor blockers should be included in the antihypertensive regimen. Recently, several clinical trials have shown the benefit of β-blockers (metoprolol and bisoprolol), α–β-blockers (carvedilol) and dihydropyridine calcium antagonists (amlodipine and felodipine), and these agents may therefore also be useful in patients with heart failure. For patients with diastolic dysfunction, non-dihydropiridone calcium antagonists, particularly verpamil, and β-blockers without intrinsic sympathomimetic activity may provide a distinct advantage over other antihypertensive agents. All drugs with negative ionotropic effects must be used with great care in patients with systolic dysfunction, especially those with class III and IV heart failure.

Other conditions

The presence of certain other comorbid conditions should also influence the choice of initial therapy for hypertension. For example:

(a) patients with bronchospasm should not be treated with β-blockers;
(b) patients with gout should not receive thiazide diuretics;
(c) elderly men with prostatism will have their blood pressure and their prostatic symptoms improved by treatment with a peripheral α-blocker;
(d) patients with renal insufficiency usually need loop-active diuretics to achieve the reduction in plasma volume that is necessary to reduce their blood pressure;
(e) patients with renal insufficiency and proteinuria from causes other than diabetes mellitus may benefit from ACE inhibitors and possibly from angiotensin receptor blockers; serum potassium must be carefully followed, although the likelihood of clinically significant hyperkalemia is small;
(f) if the clinical profile of a patient who may be a candidate for an ACE inhibitor of an angiotensin II receptor blocker suggests that there is a II reasonable probability that he or she might have unilateral or bilateral renal artery stenosis, these agents should be used only after renal artery disease has been excluded;

(g) patients with angina pectoris should be given a β-blocker or a calcium antagonist;
(h) patients who have had a recent myocardial infarction should receive a β-blocker that does not have intrinsic sympathomimetic activity, although these agents must be used with care if significant systolic dysfunction is present;
(i) patients with a low ejection fraction will almost certainly benefit from treatment with an ACE inhibitor and possibly an angiotensin II receptor blocker, and β-blockers may also be useful if used with care.
(j) cigarette smokers may not respond to non-cardioselective β-blockers that do not have intrinsic sympathomimetic activity, and so such drugs may not be appropriate;
(k) obese patients may do better with thiazide diuretics, since volume is often expanded in obesity-related hypertension;
(l) patients who wish to perform at maximum activity levels may not do well with β-blockers, and those with peripheral vascular disease or cardiac conduction defects may also be harmed by these drugs; however, patients with anxiety may be helped;
(m) non-dihydropiridine calcium antagonists and β-blockers should also be avoided in patients with cardiac conduction defects;
(n) patients with esophageal strictures or reduced esophageal motility may have problems with some sustained-released preparations; and
(o) patients with osteoporosis may do especially well with thiazide diuretics, which increase bone mass and may prevent osteoporotic fractures.

Special populations and special situations

The proper choice of initial antihypertensive therapy is also influenced by whether a patient is a member of a particular demographic subgroup. The differences in response among men and women or ethnic or age cohorts should be viewed as quantitative and not qualitative. Even though the probability of a good response to certain classes of antihypertensive agents does differ by age, ethnicity and sex, many members of all demographic groups will respond to the currently available drugs. If there are compelling or special indications for a particular drug class in a member of a subgroup in which the overall response is not as good as it is in other subgroups, he or she should still be treated with that class of agents. An individual should not be denied the potential benefit of a drug because he or she is a member of a demographic subgroup in whom the average benefit is less than that seen in other subgroups.

Demographic considerations

Blacks and other ethnic minorities
Some classes of antihypertensive agents reduce blood pressure more or less effectively in certain ethnic groups. Thiazide diuretics, for example, are more effective in blacks than whites, whereas ACE inhibitors, angiotensin II receptor blockers and β-blockers are more effective at lower doses in whites. Many blacks will respond to agents that block the renin–angiotensin–aldosterone system, but they often need higher doses than whites or Asians. However, if a black hypertensive patient would benefit from special properties that these drugs may have in type 1 diabetic patients or those with heart failure, for example, they should definitely be used even if additional agents will be needed to get blood pressure to goal. Peripheral α-blockers, α–β-blockers and calcium antagonists are equally effective in all types of hypertensive patients in all ethnic groups. In general, the response rates to antihypertensive agents in Hispanics is intermediate between that seen in whites and blacks, while East Asians, though not necessarily South Asians (patients from the Indian subcontinent), often need smaller doses than whites.

Age
All classes of antihypertensive agents lower blood pressure effectively in older persons, although the doses needed to reach goal are often lower than the doses necessary in young and middle-aged hypertensive patients. Certain drugs and certain classes of drugs, however, should be avoided or used with caution in older patients:

(a) agents such as peripheral α-blockers can exacerbate the postural fall in blood pressure that is seen more frequently in older individuals with baroreceptor dysfunction, and these agents can lead to symptomatic postural hypotension;

(b) non-dihydropyridine calcium antagonists and β-blockers may aggravate subtle or subclinical conduction defects or precipitate systolic dysfunction and heart failure, all of which are common conditions in older persons;

(c) verapamil may not be well tolerated in some older persons who are bothered by constipation;

(d) cough from ACE inhibitors may be more common in older women;

(e) in older patients with isolated systolic hypertension, diuretics may be particularly effective at lowering blood pressure, and diuretics and dihydropyridine calcium antagonists have both been shown to reduce morbidity and mortality in older persons with stage 2 or 3 isolated systolic hypertension, making them excellent choices in such patients.

Sex

There is no evidence of any difference in response to antihypertensives between men and women. The results of clinical trials in which high-risk women have been treated show that they receive the same degree of benefit as men. Concerns that women do not have the same good results with treatment as men have turned out to be groundless.

Dosage schedule

There are two elements of the dosage schedule that need to be considered when prescribing antihypertensive therapy. One is the influence of dosage schedule on the ability of patients to adhere to the regimen; the other is the need to treat hypertension for all 24 hours of the day and night.

In general, it is preferable to use drugs that are effective when given once a day. For drugs to be classified as once-a-day agents, their blood pressure-lowering effect at trough (the end of the dosing interval) should be at least 50% of their effect at peak. Some drugs formerly classified as once-a-day antihypertensive agents, such as atenolol and enalapril, may not meet these criteria and may be better used twice a day. Patients are much more likely to take their medications as prescribed if the agent is effective once or, at most, twice a day. Adherence to any therapy falls dramatically if therapy is required three times a day and if more than three pills per day of any kind are needed. All unnecessary elements of a regimen (e.g. potassium supplements or vitamins) should be stopped. Fixed-dose combinations that provide the right amounts of the desired agents can be used to reduce the number of pills taken daily and can improve adherence to the antihypertensive regimen.

Recently it has become apparent that a greater than expected percentage of myocardial infarctions, strokes and episodes of sudden cardiac death occur between 6.00 a.m. and 12.00 noon or within 1 hour of awakening.[21] One of the possible explanations as to why the early morning hours are particularly risky is the understanding that the levels of blood pressure and heart rate in both normal subjects and hypertensive patients follow a predictable circadian pattern. Blood pressure and heart rate tend to be lowest from 12.00 midnight to 4.00 a.m., at which time both begin to rise until they reach a peak at approximately 12.00 noon. They then gradually fall until 2.00 a.m. or 4.00 a.m., when, coincident with the secretion of cortisol and catecholamines, both begin to rise again. The rise in blood pressure and heart rate may predispose to the rupture of a vulnerable plaque in a coronary artery and result in a greater frequency of cardiovascular events in the morning hours.

The probable importance of the relationship between the circadian variation in hemodynamics and cardiovascular events has two important therapeutic ramifications. The first is the appreciation that blood pressure needs to be controlled for 24 hours; the other is the development of a 'chronobiological' approach to antihypertensive therapy, which is currently available only for two preparations of verapamil. These drug-delivery systems release active drug for 18–20 hours, beginning between 2.00 a.m. and 4.00 a.m., leaving the patient with no active drug in the circulation from about 10.00 p.m. to 2.00 a.m. The rationale for this approach is that blood pressure falls normally at night coincident with the usual circadian rhythm and active drug might only cause excessive lowering of the blood pressure during the middle of the night. These sustained-release preparations provide adequate active drug as the blood pressure rises before awakening and during the peak time of cardiovascular events (the period between 6.00 a.m. and 12.00 noon). The same matching of drug delivery to blood pressure is not achieved by giving 'homeostatically' designed drugs (i.e. all of the others) at night. Such agents were designed for morning use and giving them at night runs the risk of lowering blood pressure too far during sleep.

Drug interactions

The selection of initial therapy for hypertension must be done with the understanding that many hypertensive patients may not reach goal blood pressure on that agent alone and will therefore need additional antihypertensive therapy. Furthermore, many hypertensive patients need to take medications for other conditions and so the problem of drug–drug interactions is particularly pertinent.

Certain combinations of antihypertensive agents are particularly effective, such as thiazide diuretics with β-blockers, ACE inhibitors or angiotensin receptor blockers. Combinations of ACE inhibitors with calcium antagonists (both dihydropyridine and non-dihydropyridine) are also effective when used together. Dihydropyridine calcium antagonists and β-blockers are also a very effective combination, but non-dihydropyridine and β-blockers should never be used together because of the risk of excessive bradycardia and conduction defects. Thiazide diuretics are also effective with all other antihypertensive choices for double and triple therapy and with calcium antagonists. Little is known about the combination of β-blockers with central and peripheral sympatholytics and ACE inhibitors or angiotensin receptor blockers.

Most commonly used antihypertensives do not have any serious drug–drug interactions with anticoagulants, platelet inhibitors, or antibiotics. Non-dihydropyridine calcium antagonists, β-blockers and possibly telmisartan (a new angiotensin receptor blocker) must be used with care in patients who are taking digitalis preparations. Non-steroidal anti-inflammatory agents may raise blood pressure and interfere with the activity of all antihypertensive agents because of their sodium-retaining properties.

Cost

Cost considerations are now playing an increasingly important role in the pharmacological management of hypertension in the USA, and they have always been a major consideration in the rest of the world. No regimen, no matter how carefully and appropriately selected, will work if the patient cannot afford to buy it or if the agents do not appear on the national formulary or the formulary of the insurance company from whom the patient gets medication. Generic preparations are available for every class of antihypertensive agent except angiotensin receptor blockers, and these generic preparations tend to be least expensive options for initial therapy. In general, branded calcium antagonists are the most expensive, with angiotensin II receptor blockers and ACE inhibitors the next most expensive drugs. For many of the fixed-dose combinations, the cost is actually less than what would be paid for the individual components purchased separately. It is customary for those fixed-dose combinations that include a thiazide to cost no more than the non-diuretic component alone.

The real cost of antihypertensive therapy, however, is more than just the price of the drug. There are pharmacy fees to fill the prescription, which, in the USA, are the same regardless of the cost of the drug. There are office visits to evaluate the response to therapy, and blood tests to look for adverse biochemical reactions. Moreover, there is a vast potential for cost to society or individuals, if one choice of antihypertensive therapy is not as effective as others in preventing the complications of hypertension. Unfortunately, it is still not known whether newer and more expensive agents that have theoretical advantages over older and cheaper drugs would actually save money and suffering in the end, even though they are more costly at the point of service. If these drugs actually add 'value' by reducing the frequency of stroke, heart failure, myocardial infarction and end-stage renal disease more effectively than a less expensive agent, the incremental cost would be definitely worthwhile.

Mechanism of action of the drug and pathophysiology of the patient's hypertension

Some experts have felt that we could be much more successful in treating our hypertensive patients if we could tailor therapy on the basis of why the patient is hypertensive (i.e. the pathophysiologic abnormality responsible for the patient's hypertension) and could match that to the mechanism of action of the hypertensive drugs. If we knew precisely why an individual patient was hypertensive and if we could easily, safely and reliably obtain that information, treating hypertension would be relatively simple, If we really understood exactly how antihypertensive agents work, our decisions would, again, be much simpler. This approach, while intellectually appealing, has problems.

The first difficulty is that attempts to profile patients, either biochemically (e.g. by measuring plasma renin activity) or hemodynamically (e.g. by measuring cardiac output and peripheral vascular resistance) are too expensive and potentially invasive to carry out in all patients. Furthermore, these methods are not precise enough to provide the necessarily definitive information that would be needed to predict the response to therapy in a particular patient. In addition, trying to tailor therapy on the basis of the presumed pathophysiology that a group of individual patients would be expected to have is also imprecise and runs the risk of denying certain patients the potential benefits of certain classes of agents. Although it is true that blacks and older persons tend, on average, to have low or suppressed plasma renin activity, many do not. And many hypertensive patients with a low plasma renin activity will respond to drugs, such as ACE inhibitors or angiotensin II receptor blockers, that are less effective, on average, in hypertensive patients with this renin profile. In the Veterans Affairs Trial of Monotherapy, selecting initial treatment on the basis of plasma renin activity was less effective than simply using age and ethnicity (e.g. thiazide diuretics and calcium antagonists for older patients and blacks, and ACE inhibitors and β-blockers for whites and those less than 60 years of age).[22] However, neither method correctly predicted a good response in more than 63% of patients.

The second issue that complicates this approach is that many, if not all, of our drugs have more complex mechanisms of action than they were originally thought to have and work well in patient subgroups in whom they were supposed to be ineffective. For example, thiazide diuretics not only reduce plasma volume but are also vasodilators after 4 weeks of therapy. It really should not have been surprising that these agents are effective and very well tolerated in older persons even though many tend to have a modestly decreased plasma volume compared with younger hypertensive patients. Although it is true that ACE inhibitors usually suppress the endocrine renin–angiotensin–aldosterone system, the antihypertensive effect is still evident even when plasma angiotensin II levels return to pre-treatment levels. This is good evidence that there is either a tissue site of action for these drugs or that other mechanisms, perhaps the stimulation of bradykinin or nitric oxide formation, participate in how they lower blood pressure, and that the initial formulation of their mechanism of action was incomplete. It also explains why some patients with low plasma renin activity (a measure of the activity of the *endocrine* renin–angiotensin–aldosterone system) respond well to these agents or to angiotensin II receptor blockers, which suppress the renin–angiotensin–aldosterone system at the angiotensin AT_1 receptor in tissues throughout the body. Calcium antagonists were, at first, presumed to work best in older hypertensive patients and in those with suppressed plasma renin activity, but these agents are equally effective in all subgroups of hypertensives.

Perhaps the major flaw in the reasoning that we can use drugs to 'probe' the pathophysiological abnormality causing a patient's hypertension is the concept that there is only one abnormality, or one over-riding abnormality, that is responsible for a particular patient's elevated blood pressure. In all likelihood, more than one of the systems that control blood pressure, and probably many of them, are simultaneously dysfunctional, and single pharmacological agents or combinations that reduce blood pressure do so by correcting more than one abnormality.

The choice of initial therapy should be based more on other considerations than on unproven and theoretical constructs that have not turned out to be valid. However, although we cannot precisely determine the mechanism or mechanisms of action of the drugs that we use or precisely elucidate why a particular patient is hypertensive, our empiric approach to treating hypertension has dramatically reduced the rate of stroke and ischemic heart disease since we began to treat hypertension aggressively. Our approach, though far from perfect, has paid great dividends.

Summary and recommendations

Although there are numerous options and many sources of error, the successful pharmacological treatment of a hypertensive patient need not be too complicated, although neither should it be oversimplified. Once the diagnosis has been established and the routine evaluation and any more complex testing believed to be necessary are completed, lifestyle modification should begin. Lifestyle modification should be given adequate encouragement and time to work unless the patient falls in a group for which drug therapy is indicated (together with lifestyle modification) at the initiation of treatment (see *Table 4.1*). Drug therapy is indicated in all hypertensive patients if goal blood pressure is not reached with lifestyle modifications.

The following steps are recommended for choosing a regimen and then altering it until goal is reached:

(a) Deal first with cost. If the patient is unable to afford any but the least expensive drugs or cannot pay for the one that is selected, price becomes the primary issue.

(b) Ascertain whether or not other risk factors or comorbidity is present. Avoid drugs that may worsen these factors or conditions, and choose ones that might tend to improve them.

(c) Find out what clinical adverse reactions the patient whom you are treating would find the most troublesome, and avoid agents that are more likely to cause or exacerbate these problems. Some patients are not concerned at all by side effects that would be very troublesome for others.

(d) Consider demographic issues and select the class of drug with a higher probability of success, should options be available.

(e) Start with the lowest effective dose and plan to see the patient within 2–4 weeks unless the severity of the patient's hypertension or another problem warrants an earlier visit. Carry out appropriate biochemical monitoring when necessary. In some patients, start with a fixed-dose combination when it appears appropriate.

(f) Increase the dose if goal blood pressure has not been reached, even if there has been only a minimal response. Do not increase the first dose, or any dose, prematurely. Give each dose adequate time to be fully effective. If intolerable side effects occur and are likely to be drug-related, or if there has been no response, then switch to another appropriate agent for monotherapy.

(g) Continue the process of dose titration and monitoring until the maximum recommended dose has been reached. Stopping before the full dose has been reached leads to a situation in which the patient is treated with multiple agents at subtherapeutic doses when only one or two drugs is necessary.

(h) If the drug of first choice fails to reduce blood pressure to goal, add a second agent that has a different mechanism of action and that is known to have additive antihypertensive effects to the first-choice agent. A fixed-dose combination that combines two drugs in the desired doses could also be used at this time.

(i) Titrate the second drug to full dose, as was done for the first drug, and continue appropriate monitoring.

(j) Should the two-drug combination fail, consider a specific cause for the patient's refractory hypertension and, if none is evident, add a third drug, being sure that a diuretic is part of the regimen. Consider a referral to a hypertension specialist.

(k) Plan to see the patient who is at goal at least once every 3 months to be sure that blood pressure control is sustained.

(l) Reinforce the need for adherence to the regimen and always question each patient carefully about adverse reactions.

Although some patients will not reach goal with this approach even with the many effective treatment options that are available, most will come under control or close to it. Those patients who do can anticipate substantial long-term benefit with an extended life expectancy and a much reduced risk of stroke, ischemic heart disease, heart failure and probably renal failure and dementia.

Although treating high blood pressure can be costly and at times seemingly unrewarding, the benefits to individual patients and to society make the effort worthwhile. We must be careful not to become apathetic about hypertension. The problem is not solved, and it will not be solved until all hypertensive patients are able to avail themselves of what has been among the most successful examples of preventive medicine.

References

1. Murray CJ, Lopez AD. Evidence-based health policy: lessons from the Global Burden of Disease Study. Science 1999; 274: 740–743.

2. The Sixth Report of the Joint National Committee on Prevention, Detection, Evaluation, and treatment of High Blood Pressure. Arch Intern Med 1997; 157: 2413–2446.

3. Staessen JA, Fagard R, Thijs L *et al.* for the Systolic Hypertension Europe Syst-Eur Trial Investigators. Morbidity and mortality in the placebo-controlled European Trial on Isolated Systolic Hypertension in the Elderly. Lancet 1997; 350: 757–764.

4. Hansson L, Lindholm LH, Niskanen L *et al.* Effect of angiotensin-converting-enzyme inhibition compared with conventional therapy on cardiovascular morbidity and mortality in hypertension: the Captopril Prevention Project (CAPPP) randomized trial. Lancet 1999; 353: 611–616.

5. World Health Organization. International Society of Hypertension Blood Pressure Lowering Treatment Trialists' Collaboration: protocol for prospective collaborative overviews of major randomized trials of blood-pressure-lowering treatments. J Hypertens 1998; 16: 127–138.

6. Davis BR, Cutler JA, Gordon DJ *et al.* Rationale and design for the Antihypertensive and Lipid Lowering Treatment to prevent Heart Attack Trial (ALLHAT). Am J Hypertens 1996; 9: 342–360.

7. Black HR, Elliott WJ, Neaton JD. Rationale and design for the Controlled ONset Verapamil INvestigation of Cardiovascular Endpoints (CONVINCE) trial. Controlled Clin Trials 1998; 19: 370–390.

8. 1999 World Health Organization–International Society of Hypertension Guidelines for the Management of Hypertension. Guidelines Subcommittee. J Hypertens 1999; 17: 151–183.

9. Hansson L, Zanchetti A, Julius S *et al.* Effects of intensive blood pressure lowering and low-dose aspirin in patients with hypertension: principal results of the Hypertension Optimal Treatment (HOT) randomised trial. Lancet 1998; 351: 1755–1762.

10. UK Prospective Diabetes Study Group. Tight blood pressure control and risk of macrovascular and microvascular complications in type 2 diabetes: UKPDS 38. BMJ 1998; 317: 703–713.

11. Elliott WJ, Weir DR, Black HR. Cost-effectiveness of the lower treatment goal of JNC VI for diabetic hypertensives. Arch Intern Med; in press.

12. Ramsay LE, Williams B, Johnston GD *et al.* Guidelines for management of hypertension: report of the third working party of the British Hypertension Society. J Hum Hypertens 1999; 13: 569–592.

13. Black HR. Metabolic considerations in the choice of therapy for the hypertensive patient. Am Heart J 1991; 121: 707–715.

14. Curb JD, Pressel SL, Cutler J *et al.* Effect of diuretic-based antihypertensive treatment on cardiovascular disease risk in older diabetics with isolated systolic hypertension. JAMA 1996; 276: 1886–1892.

15. Lewis EJ, Hunsicker LG, Bain RP, Rohde RD. The effect of angiotensin-converting-enzyme inhibition on diabetic nephropathy. The Collaborative Study Group. N Engl J Med 1993; 329: 1456–1462.

16. Tuomilehto J, Rastenyte D, Birkenhager WH *et al.* Effects of calcium-channel blockade in older patients with diabetes and systolic hypertension. Systolic Hypertension in Europe Trial Investigators. N Engl J Med 1999; 340: 677–684.

17. Dahlöf B, Pennert K, Hansson L. Reversal of left ventricular hypertrophy in hypertensive patients. A metaanalysis of 109 treatment studies. Am J Hypertens 1992; 5: 95–110.

18. Schmieder RE, Martus P, Klingbeil A. Reversal of left ventricular hypertrophy in essential hypertension. A meta-analysis of randomized double-blind studies. JAMA 1996; 275: 1507–1513.

19. Neaton JD, Grimm RH Jr, Prineas RJ *et al.* Treatment of Mild Hypertension Study. Final results. Treatment of Mild Hypertension Study Research Group. JAMA 1993; 270: 713–724.

20. Materson BJ, Reda DJ, Cushman WC *et al.* Single-drug therapy for hypertension in men. A comparison of six antihypertensive agents with placebo. The Department of Veterans Affairs Cooperative Study Group on Antihypertensive Agents. N Engl J Med 1993; 328: 914–924.

21. Muller JE. Circadian variation in cardiovascular events. Am J Hypertens 1999; 12: 35S–42S.

22. Preston RA, Materson BJ, Reda DJ *et al.* for the Department of Veterans Affairs Cooperative Study Group on Antihypertensive Agents. Age–race subgroup compared with renin profile as predictors of blood pressure response to antihypertensive therapy. JAMA 1999; 280: 1168–1172.

5
Clinical trials in older patients with systolic hypertension

Jan A Staessen

Introduction

Systolic blood pressure increases with age at least until the eighth decade of life.[1,2] In contrast, diastolic blood pressure rises only until middle age and in older subjects either levels off or even slightly decreases. These divergent trends in systolic and diastolic blood pressure have been observed in cross-sectional studies[1,2] as well as in longitudinal studies[1] and explain why pulse pressure and the prevalence of isolated systolic hypertension rise with advancing age. In Western countries, the isolated systolic hypertension occurs in around 15% of men and women aged 60 years or more; in octagenarians its prevalence even exceeds 20% (*Fig. 5.1*). Isolated systolic hypertension is largely due to a decrease in the elasticity of the large arteries and is not necessarily accompanied by a rise in mean arterial blood pressure or peripheral resistance.[3]

In the elderly, systolic hypertension is the most important cardiovascular risk factor amenable to intervention.[3] In some reports[4] the hypothesis has been put forward that the excess cardiovascular risk of hypertensive patients, compared with age-matched normotensive controls, decreases as the age of onset of high blood pressure is more advanced. However, this point of view is contradicted by the evidence from numerous cross-sectional and longitudinal observational studies[3] as well as by the results of the outcome trials in older hypertensive patients.[5] The predominance of systolic over diastolic blood pressure as a cardiovascular risk indicator in the elderly is not just an artefact, because of the larger range of systolic blood pressure. This observation still stands, if systolic and diastolic blood pressures are expressed on a standardized scale in units of standard deviation.

The ultimate goal of treating elderly patients with hypertension is not to reduce their blood pressure but to prevent the cardiovascular complications of hypertension, so that longevity increases and quality of life improves. Three placebo-controlled outcome trials on antihypertensive drug treatment of isolated systolic hypertension have been published: the

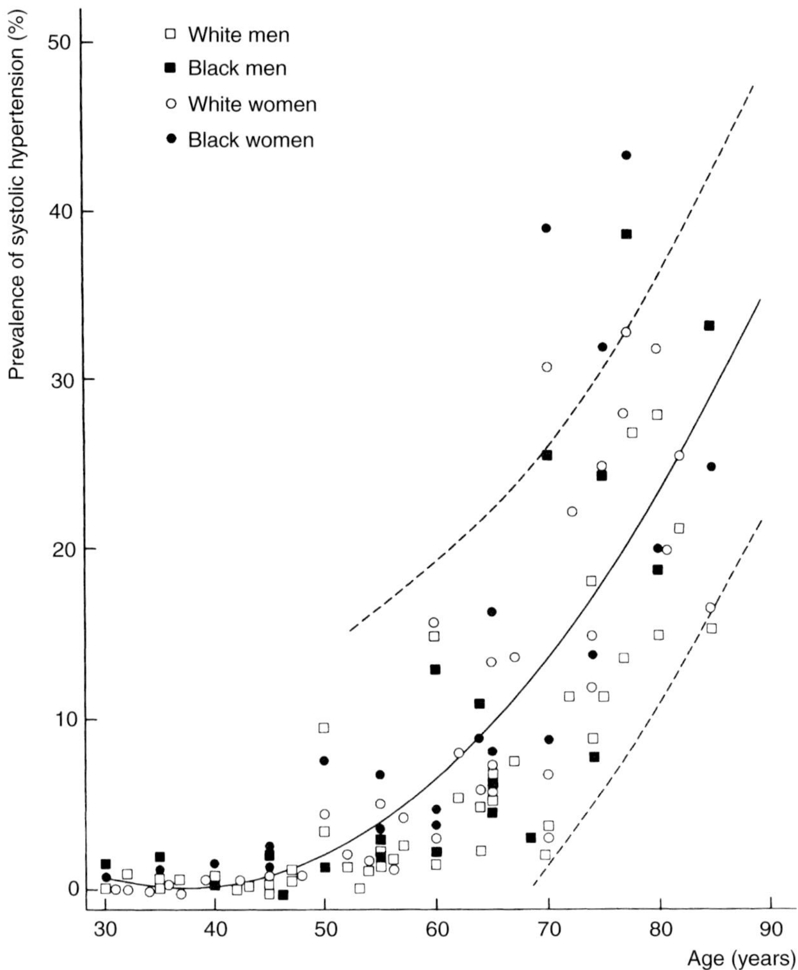

Figure 5.1

Prevalence of isolated systolic hypertension by the mid-point of the age classes reported in various studies. As shown by the regression line (unweighted), the prevalence of systolic hypertension rises curvilinearly with age. The 95% CI for the prediction of individual points is presented for the age range from 50 to 90 years. From Staessen et al.,[3] with permission.

Systolic Hypertension in the Elderly Program (SHEP),[6] the Systolic Hypertension in Europe (Syst-Eur) trial,[7] and the Systolic Hypertension in China (Syst-China) trial.[8] The main results of these three studies were published in 1991, 1997, and 1998 respectively and will be reviewed in this chapter.

The SHEP trial

The SHEP investigators were the first to complete an outcome trial of anti-hypertensive drug treatment in older patients with isolated systolic hypertension.[6,9] A total of 4736 patients (1.1%) from 447,921 patients screened, aged 60 years or above, were randomized to active treatment (n = 2365) or placebo (n = 2371). Systolic blood pressure ranged from 160 to 219 mmHg and diastolic blood pressure was <90 mmHg. The average blood pressure at entry was 170 mmHg systolic and 77 mmHg diastolic. Mean age was 72 years. Of the participants, 57% were female, 14% were black and 33% had previously been treated for hypertension. Before randomization, the patients were stratified by clinical center and by antihypertensive treatment status at initial contact. Active treatment was started with the thiazide diuretic chlorthalidone (12.5–25 mg per day) with the possible addition of atenolol (25–50 mg per day). In patients with known contraindications for atenolol, the β-blocker could be replaced by reserpine (0.05–0.1 mg per day). Matching placebos were used in a similar fashion in the placebo group.

Main morbidity and mortality results

Follow-up averaged 4.5 years. The 5-year systolic/diastolic blood pressure averaged 155/72 mmHg in the placebo group and 143/68 mmHg in the active-treatment group. Active treatment reduced total stroke incidence from 16.4 to 10.4 events per 1000 patient–years (−36%; 95% confidence interval (CI) −50 to −18%; $p < 0.001$). Drug treatment also decreased non-fatal stroke by 37% (CI 18–51%), non-fatal myocardial infarction by 33% (CI 4–53%), non-fatal myocardial infarction combined with coronary death by 27% (CI 6–43%), non-fatal left ventricular failure by 54% (CI 35–67%), and all major cardiovascular complications by 32% (CI 21–42%). Total mortality was not significantly influenced (−13%; CI −27 to +5%). The 5-year absolute benefit with regard to stroke and major cardiovascular end-points amounted to 30 and 55 prevented events per 1000 treated participants,[6] respectively, and was equally observed in all stratification groups.[6,9]

Outcome in diabetic and non-diabetic patients

At baseline, 583 SHEP patients (12.3%) had non-insulin-dependent diabetes mellitus, 4149 patients did not have diabetes, and four patients could not be classified.[10] In the SHEP control group, the rate of all cardiovascular complications was 63.0 events per 1000 patient–years in the diabetic patients (n = 300) and 36.8 events per 1000 patient–years in the group without diabetes (n = 2069); in the diabetic patients (n = 283) and the non-diabetic patients (n = 2080) who were randomized to active

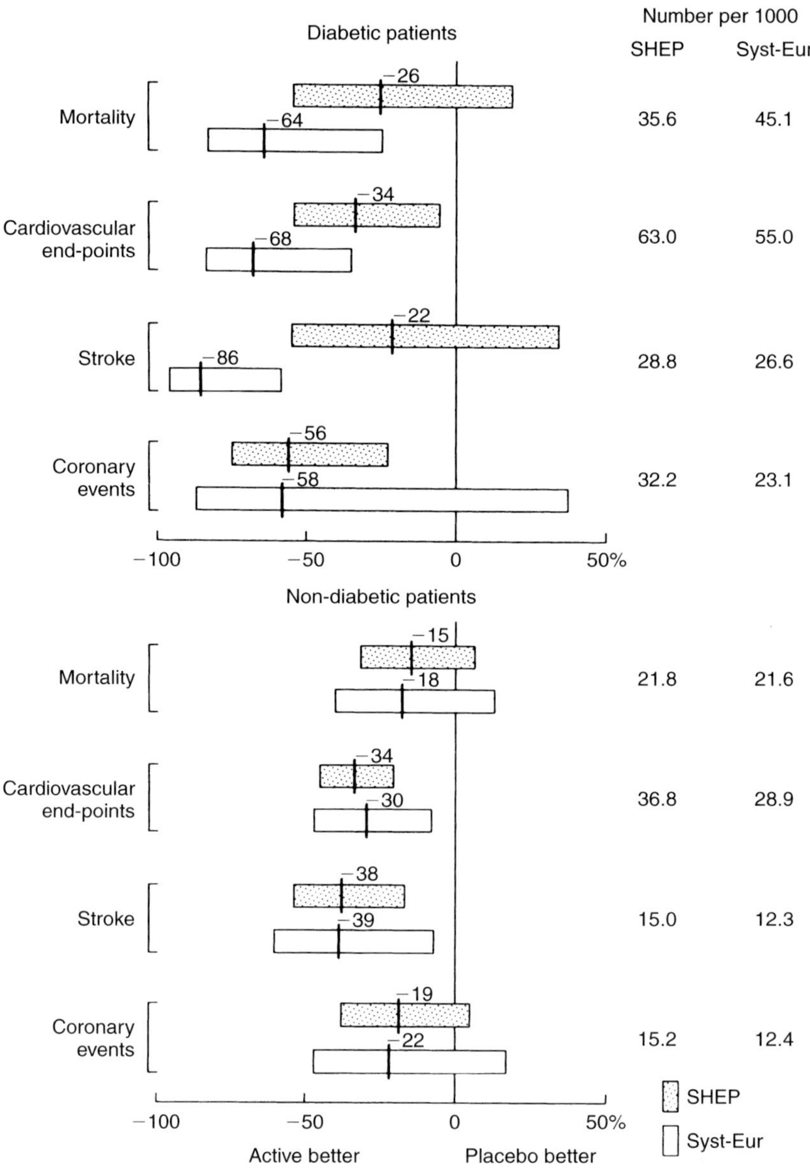

Figure 5.2

Outcome results in the diabetic and non-diabetic patients randomized in the SHEP[10] and Syst-Eur[11] trials. For this analysis the end-points were standardized to the definitions used in the SHEP trial.[10] The changes with active treatment were calculated by Cox regression with adjustments applied for sex, age, smoking, systolic and diastolic blood pressure at baseline, electrocardiographic abnormalities (SHEP) or previous cardiovascular complications (Syst-Eur) at baseline, and race (SHEP) or residence in western Europe (Syst-Eur). From Tuomilehto *et al.*,[11] with permission.

treatment, these rates were reduced to 42.8 and 26.6 events per 1000 patient–years, respectively.[10] Thus, in the SHEP trial (*Fig. 5.2*), active treatment decreased the incidence of all cardiovascular complications to the same extent (−34%) in diabetics (CI −54 to −6%) and non-diabetics (CI −45 to −21%).[10]

Incidence of dementia

During the course of the SHEP trial, about 4% of persons in the active-treatment and placebo groups met questionnaire referral criteria for expert evaluation of possible dementia. For more than 90% of these people a referral was completed; the main reason for failure to achieve referral was refusal of the participant. The overall incidence of dementia was low and similar in the two treatment groups: 37% participants (1.6%) who were receiving active treatment and 44 (1.9%) who were receiving placebo had a diagnosis of dementia made and confirmed by the coding panel (*Fig. 5.3*).

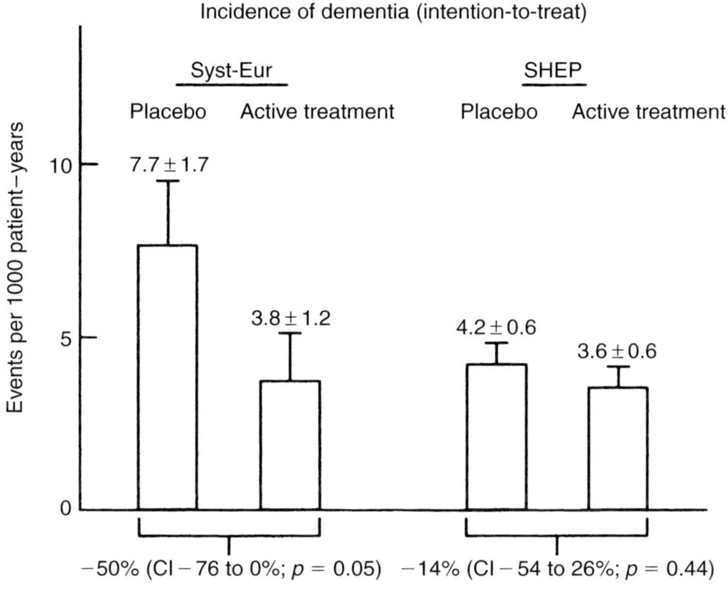

Figure 5.3

Incidence of dementia in the intention-to-treat analysis of the SHEP[6] and Syst-Eur[24] trials. The SHEP results were calculated from the data published by SHEP Cooperative Research Group.[6]

The Syst-Eur trial

In 1989, the European Working Party on High Blood Pressure in the Elderly initiated the double-blind placebo-controlled Syst-Eur trial.[7,12,13] In view of the remaining uncertainties with regard to the treatment of isolated systolic hypertension in the elderly,[14–18] this trial continued after the publication of the SHEP results.[6] Furthermore, the recent controversy about the role of calcium channel blockers as first-line antihypertensive agents[19,20] highlighted the lack of evidence that this newer class of drugs could reduce cardiovascular risk.

As in the SHEP study,[6,9] patients who were eligible for enrollment in the Syst-Eur trial[7,11] were at least 60 years old. At three run-in visits 1 month apart, their sitting systolic blood pressure on single-blind placebo treatment averaged from 160 to 219 mmHg with diastolic blood pressure lower than 95 mmHg. Of the participants, 67% were female and 47% had previously been treated for hypertension.[7] After stratification for center, sex, and previous cardiovascular complications, 4695 patients were randomized. Active treatment consisted of nitrendipine (10–40 mg per day) with the possible addition of enalapril (5–20 mg per day) and/or hydrochlorothiazide (12.5–25 mg per day), titrated or combined to reduce the sitting systolic blood pressure by at least 20 mmHg to below 150 mmHg. Matching placebo tablets were employed similarly. Patients who withdrew from double-blind treatment were followed further to facilitate the intention-to-treat analysis.[7]

Main morbidity and mortality results in the intention-to-treat analysis

At 2 years (median follow-up) the sitting blood pressure had fallen by 13/2 mmHg in the placebo group (n = 2297) and by 23/7 mmHg in the active-treatment group (n = 2398). The between-group blood pressure differences were 10.1 mmHg systolic (CI 8.8–11.4 mmHg) and 4.5 mmHg diastolic (CI 3.9–5.1 mmHg).

Cardiovascular mortality tended to be less on active treatment (−27%; CI −48 to 2%; $p = 0.07$), but all-cause mortality was not significantly changed (*Table 5.1*). In the placebo group the mortality rate due to stroke, heart failure, myocardial infarction, or sudden death ranged from 1.8 to 4.7 deaths per 1000 patient–years. Although mortality from these causes was less for the patients on active treatment, the CIs of these changes were wide and did not exclude the possibility of no effect of antihypertensive drug treatment. Non-cardiovascular and cancer mortality did not change significantly (see *Table 5.1*).

As shown in *Table 5.2*, active treatment reduced the total stroke rate from 13.7 to 7.9 events per 1000 patient–years (−42% CI: −60 to −17%; $p = 0.003$). Non-fatal stroke alone decreased by 44% (CI 14–63%; $p = 0.007$). In the active-treatment group, all fatal and non-fatal cardiac

Table 5.1 Mortality by treatment group in the intention-to-treat analysis of the Syst-Eur trial[7]

Cause of death	Rate per 1000 patient–years (number of deaths)		Relative difference with rate in placebo group	
	Placebo (n = 2297)	Active (n = 2398)	% rate (95% CI)	p
All causes	24.0 (137)	20.5 (123)	−14 (−33, 9)	0.22
Unknown cause	0.4 (2)	0.7 (4)	—	—
Cardiovascular causes	13.5 (77)	9.8 (59)	−27 (−48 to +2)	0.07
Stroke	3.7 (21)	2.7 (16)	−27 (−62 to +39)	0.33
Cardiac mortality*	9.1 (52)	6.7 (40)	−27 (−51 to +11)	0.14
Heart failure	1.8 (10)	1.3 (8)	−24 (−70 to +93)	0.57
Coronary mortality†	7.4 (42)	5.3 (32)	−27 (−54 to +15)	0.17
Myocardial infarction	2.6 (15)	1.2 (7)	−56 (−82 to +9)	0.08
Sudden death	4.7 (27)	4.2 (25)	−12 (−49 to +52)	0.65
Dissecting aortic aneurysm	0.4 (2)	0.2 (1)	—	—
Pulmonary embolism	0.2 (1)	0.3 (2)	—	—
Peripheral arterial disease	0.2 (1)	0.0 (0)	—	—
Non-cardiovascular causes	10.2 (58)	10.0 (60)	−1 (−31 to +41)	0.95
Cancer	4.4 (25)	3.0 (18)	−31 (−63 to +26)	0.22

*Cardiac mortality included deaths from heart failure and coronary mortality.
†Coronary mortality consisted of fatal myocardial infarction and sudden death.

end-points, including sudden death, declined by 26% (CI 3–44%; $p = 0.03$). Non-fatal cardiac end-points decreased by 33% (CI 3–53%; $p = 0.03$). Similar trends were also observed (see *Table 5.2*) for non-fatal heart failure (−36%; CI −60 to +2%; $p = 0.06$), for all cases of heart failure (−29%; CI −53 to +10%; $p = 0.12$), and for fatal and non-fatal myocardial infarction (−30%; CI −56 to +9%; $p = 0.12$). Active treatment reduced all fatal and non-fatal cardiovascular end-points by 31% (CI 14–45%; $p<0.001$). Treating 1000 patients for 5 years could prevent 29 strokes or 53 major cardiovascular events.

Other morbidity and mortality results

In subgroup analyses,[13] active treatment was equally beneficial in all stratification groups. Furthermore, the benefit of antihypertensive drug treatment on total ($p = 0.009$) and cardiovascular ($p = 0.09$) mortality weakened with advancing age, suggesting that in very old patients (those aged 80 years or over) only non-fatal end-points were prevented. The trend towards a reduction of total mortality on active treatment also decreased ($p = 0.05$) with lower systolic blood pressure at entry. For fatal and nonfatal stroke, the benefit of active treatment ($p = 0.01$) was evident only in non-smokers (92.5% of all patients).

Benefit was equally noticed in patients who remained on monotherapy with active nitrendipine.[21] In a matched-pair analysis, 1327 patients who continued monotherapy with active nitrendipine were matched by sex, age (60–69 years, 70–79 years, and 80 years or over), previous cardiovascular complications, and systolic blood pressure at entry (within 4 mmHg) with an equal number of patients drawn from the control group, regardless of the type and the number of placebo tablets taken. At 2 years (median follow-up in the two groups), the net blood pressure reduction in the actively treated patients averaged 13.7 mmHg systolic (CI 11.9–15.5 mmHg) and 5.4 mmHg diastolic (CI 4.5–6.4 mmHg). Compared with the matched control group, active nitrendipine reduced cardiovascular mortality by 41% (CI 0–66%; $p = 0.05$), all cardiovascular end-points by 33% (CI 8–51%; $p = 0.01$), fatal and non-fatal cardiac end-points by 33% (CI 0–55%; $p = 0.05$), and fatal and non-fatal heart failure by 48% (CI 0–73%; $p = 0.05$).[21]

The per-protocol analysis of the Syst-Eur trial[13] considered only the end-points that had occurred during double-blind treatment and confirmed the results obtained in the intention-to-treat analysis.[7] However, in the per-protocol analysis,[13] active treatment also decreased total mortality by 26% (CI 0–46%; $p = 0.05$). The per-protocol analysis suggested that treating 1000 patients for 5 years could prevent 24 deaths, 54 major cardiovascular end-points, 29 strokes, or 25 cardiac end-points.

Table 5.2 Non-fatal end-points alone and combined with fatal end-points in the intention-to-treat analysis of the Syst-Eur trial[7]

Nature of end-point	Rate per 1000 patient–years (number of end-points)		Relative difference with rate in placebo group	
	Placebo (n = 2297)	Active (n = 2398)	% rate (95% CI)	p
Non-fatal end-points				
Stroke	10.1 (57)	5.7 (34)	−44 (−63, −14)	0.007
Retinal exudates	0.0 (0)	0.2 (1)	—	—
Cardiac end-points	12.6 (70)	8.5 (50)	−33 (−53 to −3)	0.03
Heart failure	7.6 (43)	4.9 (29)	−36 (−60 to +2)	0.06
Myocardial infarction	5.5 (31)	4.4 (26)	−20 (−53 to +34)	0.40
Renal failure	0.4 (2)	0.5 (3)	—	—
Fatal and non-fatal end-points				
Stroke	13.7 (77)	7.9 (47)	−42 (−60 to −17)	0.003
Cardiac end-points*	20.5 (114)	15.1 (89)	−26 (−44 to −3)	0.03
Heart failure	8.7 (49)	6.2 (37)	−29 (−53 to +10)	0.12
Myocardial infarction	8.0 (45)	5.5 (33)	−30 (−56 to +9)	0.12
All cardiovascular end-points	33.9 (186)	23.3 (137)	−31 (−45 to −14)	<0.001

*Non-fatal and fatal cardiac end-points included fatal and non-fatal heart failure, fatal and non-fatal myocardial infarction, and sudden death (see *Table 5.1*).

Outcome in diabetic and non-diabetic patients

Of the 4695 randomized Syst-Eur patients, 492 (10.5%) had diabetes mellitus at entry.[11] Compared with the 4203 non-diabetic patients, the diabetic patients had higher systolic blood pressure (175.3 mmHg versus 173.7 mmHg), lower diastolic blood pressure (84.5 mmHg versus 85.6 mmHg), higher mean blood glucose concentrations (8.2 mmol/l versus 5.1 mmol/l), higher body mass index (28.3 kg/m^2 versus 27 kg/m^2), and lower high-density lipoprotein cholesterol concentrations (1.3 mmol/l versus 1.4 mmol/l).[11] A significantly greater proportion of the diabetic patients had experienced cardiovascular complications before enrollment and their rate of cardiovascular complications during the trial was about twice the rate that was observed in the non-diabetic patients.

Active treatment significantly reduced cardiovascular complications in the diabetic patients (*Fig. 5.4*). After controlling for possible confounders, total mortality was reduced by 55% (CI 15–76%), cardiovascular mortality by 76% (CI 33–91%), all cardiovascular end-points by 69% (CI 41–84%), fatal and non-fatal stroke by 73% (CI 26–90%), and all cardiac end-points by 63% (CI 10–85%). In the non-diabetic patients, active treatment decreased all cardiovascular end-points by 26% (CI 6–41%) and fatal and non-fatal stroke by 38% (CI 8–58%). Active treatment reduced total mortality, cardiovascular mortality and all cardiovascular end-points significantly more in the diabetic patients than in the non-diabetic patients (*p*-values 0.04, 0.02, and 0.01, respectively). Thus, the dihydropyridine-based treatment was particularly effective in diabetic patients, in whom active treatment was estimated to prevent 178 severe cardiovascular complications as opposed to only 22 in the non-diabetic group.[11]

Prevention of Alzheimer's disease

The Vascular Dementia Project[22–24] investigated whether antihypertensive drug treatment could reduce the incidence of dementia. At baseline and follow-up, cognitive function was assessed by the mini-mental state examination;[25] if the score was 23 or less, the diagnosis of dementia was established on the basis of the DSM-III-R criteria.[26] In total, 2418 patients were enrolled in the dementia study. Median follow-up by intention to treat was 2.0 years.

Among the 32 incident cases of dementia, 23 were Alzheimer's disease, seven had a mixed etiology, and only two were vascular. Compared with placebo (n = 1180), active treatment (n = 1238) reduced the incidence of dementia by 50% (CI 0–76%; *p* = 0.05) from 7.7 down to 3.8 cases per 1000 patient–years (*Fig. 5.3*). At the risk observed in the placebo group, treating 1000 hypertensive patients for 5 years could prevent 19 dementia cases. In the per-protocol analysis, active treatment decreased the rate by 60% (CI 2–83%; *p* = 0.03). Thus, active treatment prevented mainly Alzheimer's disease.

Table 5.3 Update on the morbidity and mortality results in the intention-to-treat analysis of the Syst-Eur trial[27]

Nature of end-point	Rate per 1000 patient–years (number of end-points)		Relative difference with rate in placebo group	
	Placebo (n = 2297)	Active (n = 2398)	% rate (95% CI)	p
Mortality				
Total	25.2 (147)	22.0 (135)	−13 (−31 to +10)	0.28
Cardiovascular	14.0 (82)	10.4 (64)	−26 (−46 to +3)	0.08
Non-cardiovascular	11.0 (64)	10.8 (66)	−2 (−30 to +38)	0.94
Non-fatal end-points				
Stroke	10.4 (60)	5.7 (35)	−45 (−64 to −17)	0.004
Cardiac end-points	12.8 (73)	8.8 (53)	−32 (−52 to −2)	0.04
Fatal and non-fatal end-points				
Stroke	13.9 (80)	8.0 (49)	−42 (−60 to −18)	0.002
Cardiac end-points*	20.9 (119)	15.6 (94)	−25 (−43 to −2)	0.03
Heart failure	8.9 (51)	6.6 (40)	−26 (−51 to +12)	0.16
Myocardial infarction	8.1 (47)	5.9 (36)	−27 (−53 to +12)	0.16
All cardiovascular end-points	34.6 (194)	24.2 (145)	−30 (−44 to −13)	<0.001

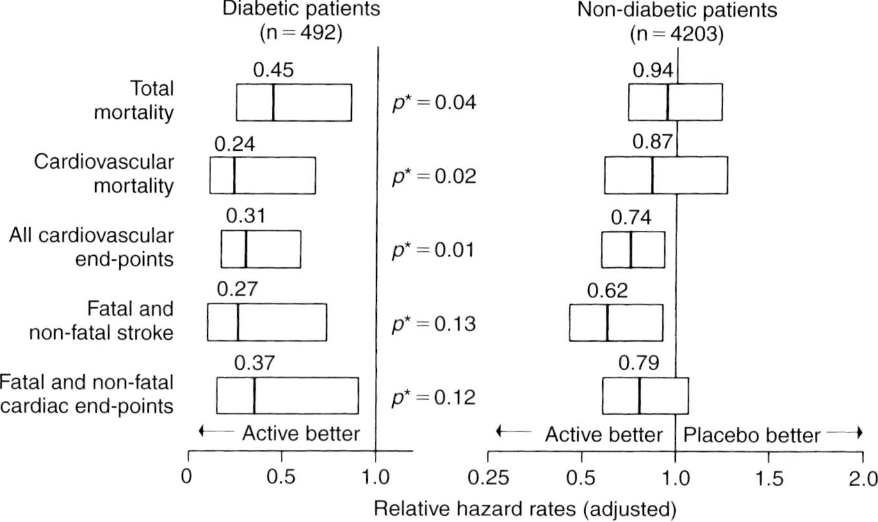

Figure 5.4

Relative hazard rates of active treatment *vs* placebo in diabetic and non-diabetic patients with cumulative adjustments for sex, age, previous cardiovascular complications, systolic blood pressure at entry, smoking, and residence in western Europe. The *p* values refer to the treatment-by-diabetes interaction and indicate whether the treatment effect was significantly different according to the presence of diabetes at randomization. This analysis is based on the Syst-Eur definitions of end-points.[7] (*p value for interaction between active treatment and diabetes). From Tuomilehto *et al.*,[11] with permission.

Update on the morbidity and mortality results

The Syst-Eur trial stopped after the second of four planned interim analyses, when predefined stopping rules[12] revealed that active treatment diminished the incidence of stroke, the primary end-point. The ethics committee unanimously resolved that all end-points that had occurred before 14 February 1997, at 5.00 p.m. should be included in the final analysis. The long communication lines between the co-ordinating office and the 198 centres in 23 countries made the practical implementation of this recommendation very difficult. The co-ordinating office had to strike a delicate balance between reporting long-awaited outcome results and postponing publication until a greater number of terminating report forms had been returned. In the initial Syst-Eur report (see *Tables 5.1* and *5.2*),[7] 116 (5.1%) of the 2297 placebo patients and 121 (5.0%) of the 2398 patients randomized to active treatment were classified as lost to follow-up, because in the preceeding year no report had reached the co-ordinating office. However, after publication of the outcome results on 13

September 1997,[7] efforts to locate all patients continued and the database was updated.[27]

The number of patients lost to follow-up decreased to 61 (2.7%) in the placebo group and to 63 (2.6%) in the active-treatment group—1559 and 1795 patients, respectively, were in double-blind follow-up, 147 and 135 had died, 283 and 150 were in supervised open follow-up, and 247 and 255 were in non-supervised follow-up.[27] The number of patient-years accumulated in the placebo and active-treatment groups increased from 5709 to 5844 and from 5995 to 6140, respectively. The greater number of end-points available for analysis (*Table 5.3*) did not affect the conclusions of the initial Syst-Eur report (see *Tables 5.1* and *5.2*).[7] Fatal and non-fatal cancer (change with active treatment: -12%; CI -36 to $+20\%$; $p = 0.42$) and bleeding episodes not including cerebral and retinal hemorrhage (-9%; CI -50 to 65%; $p = 0.96$) occurred with similar frequency in both treatment groups.

Ambulatory blood pressure as a cardiovascular risk factor

The Syst-Eur trial was the first large-scale outcome trial in hypertension in which ambulatory blood pressure recordings were obtained in a substantial proportion of the randomized patients.[28–30] Follow-up of the placebo group also gave the possibility of validating proposed diagnostic thresholds[31,32] for blood pressure monitoring in terms of morbidity and mortality. Of the 198 Syst-Eur centers, 46 opted to enroll their patients, and for 808 Syst-Eur patients a baseline ambulatory blood pressure recording of sufficient quality was available.

Systolic blood pressure was on average 22.0 mmHg higher ($p < 0.001$) on conventional than on ambulatory measurement than it was on daytime ambulatory measurement; diastolic blood pressure was on average 2.0 mmHg higher ($p < 0.001$) (*Table 5.4*). The corresponding mean ± 2 SD intervals ranged from -8.3 to $+52.3$ mmHg and from -17.2 to $+21.2$ mmHg, respectively. Awake and sleeping blood pressures were similar to daytime (from 10.00 a.m. to 8.00 p.m.) and night-time (from midnight to 6.00 a.m.) blood pressures. The results of Cox regression were also similar, regardless of which of the two definitions of the diurnal high and low blood pressure spans was considered. Because short, fixed-clocktime intervals[33] are easy to reproduce across studies, only the results for the daytime and the night-time blood pressures were reported. The mean (SD) within-subject coefficient of variation was significantly smaller for the night-time blood pressure than for the daytime blood pressure (8.7 (3.6)% versus 10.4 (3.3)%; $p < 0.001$).

With cumulative adjustments applied for sex, age, previous cardiovascular complications, smoking, and residence in western Europe,[13] a higher systolic blood pressure at randomization predicted a worse prognosis, whereas the association between diastolic blood pressure and

Table 5.4 Conventional and ambulatory blood pressures at randomization in 808 Syst-Eur patients[30]

	Mean (SD) systolic blood pressure (mmHg)	Mean (SD) diastolic, blood pressure (mmHg)
Conventional* blood pressure in the sitting position	173.3 (10.8)	86.0 (5.8)
Ambulatory blood pressure		
24-hour	145.8 (15.6)	79.3 (8.9)
Daytime (10.00 a.m. to 8.00 p.m.)	151.4 (16.2)	84.1 (9.8)
Night-time (midnight to 6.00 a.m.)	134.0 (18.6)	70.2 (10.1)
Nocturnal blood pressure fall†	17.4 (14.8)	13.8 (8.8)
Night-to-day blood pressure ratio‡	0.89 (0.09)	0.84 (0.10)
Awake	151.0 (15.8)	83.6 (9.4)
Sleeping	134.7 (18.1)	70.8 (9.9)

*Mean of six readings, i.e., two at each of three baseline visits 1 month apart.

†Daytime minus night-time blood pressure.

‡Dimensionless ratio of night-time to daytime blood pressure.

outcome was not significant. In the placebo group (n = 393), the 24-hour, daytime, and night-time systolic ambulatory blood pressures predicted the incidence of cardiovascular complications even after further adjustment for the conventional blood pressure (*Table 5.5*). The night-time systolic blood pressure behaved as a more accurate predictor of end-points (except stroke) than the daytime level. The 24-hour level and the night-to-day ratio of systolic blood pressure were significantly and independently correlated with the incidence of all cardiovascular end-points in the placebo group. The relative hazard rates associated with a 10 mmHg increase in the 24-hour blood pressure and with a 10% higher night-to-day ratio were 1.23 (CI 1.03–1.46; *p* = 0.02) and 1.41 (CI 1.03–1.94; *p* = 0.03), respectively. In the placebo group, the cardiovascular risk conferred by a conventional systolic blood pressure of 160 mmHg at randomization was similar to risks associated with a 24-hour, daytime, or night-time systolic blood pressure of 142 mmHg (CI 128–156 mmHg), 145 mmHg (CI 126–164 mmHg) or 132 mmHg (CI 120–145 mmHg), respectively. In the active-treatment group (n = 415), systolic blood pressure at randomization did not significantly predict cardiovascular risk, regardless of the technique of blood pressure measurement.

The Syst-China trial

Isolated systolic hypertension occurs in around 8% of Chinese people aged 60 years or older.[34] In 1988, the Syst-China Collaborative Group started to investigate whether active treatment could reduce the incidence of stroke and other cardiovascular complications in older patients with isolated systolic hypertension.[8,34,35] All patients were initially started on placebo. After stratification for center, sex, and previous cardiovascular complications, patients (n = 1253) were alternate assigned sequentially to receive nitrendipine 10–40 mg daily, with the possible addition of captopril 12.5–50.0 mg daily, hydrochlorothiazide 12.5–50.0 mg daily, or both drugs. These study medications were titrated or combined to reduce the sitting systolic blood pressure by at least 20 mmHg to below 150 mmHg. In the remaining 1141 control patients, matching placebos were employed similarly.

Main morbidity and mortality results

At entry, sitting blood pressure averaged 170 mmHg systolic and 86 mmHg diastolic. The average age was 66.5 years. The average total serum cholesterol was 5.1 mmol/l.[8] At 2 years of follow-up, the sitting systolic and diastolic blood pressures had fallen by 11 mmHg and 2 mmHg in the placebo group and by 20 mmHg and 5 mmHg in the active-treatment group. The between-group differences were 9.1 mmHg systolic (CI 7.6–10.7 mmHg) and 3.2 mmHg diastolic (CI 2.4–4.0 mmHg).

Table 5.5 Relative hazard rates* for ambulatory systolic blood pressure after adjustment for the conventional systolic blood pressure and various entry characteristics[30]

	Mortality		Fatal and non-fatal end-points combined		
	Total	Cardiovascular causes	Cardiovascular	Stroke	Cardiac
Placebo group (n = 393)					
24-hour blood pressure	1.19 (0.95–1.49)	1.29 (0.95–1.75)	1.27 (1.05–1.54)‡	1.51 (1.06–2.15)‡	1.14 (0.90–1.43)
Daytime blood pressure	1.14 (0.91–1.42)	1.25 (0.92–1.69)	1.20 (1.00–1.45)‡	1.61 (1.14–2.28)§	1.06 (0.85–1.33)
Night-time blood pressure	1.21 (1.00–1.47)‡	1.39 (1.07–1.79)‡	1.31 (1.12–1.53)¶	1.25 (0.94–1.66)	1.22 (1.06–1.54)‡
Active treatment (n = 415)					
24-hour blood pressure	0.95 (0.72–1.24)	0.89 (0.61–1.30)	1.05 (0.84–1.31)	1.15 (0.69–1.90)	1.05 (0.81–1.35)
Daytime blood pressure	0.81 (0.62–1.06)	0.86 (0.60–1.25)	0.94 (0.77–1.16)	0.82 (0.52–1.29)	0.97 (0.77–1.24)
Night-time blood pressure	1.05 (0.86–1.27)	1.00 (0.77–1.30)	1.12 (0.95–1.32)	1.38 (0.96–2.00)	1.07 (0.89–1.29)
Both groups (n = 808)‖					
24-hour blood pressure	1.09 (0.92–1.29)	1.11 (0.88–1.40)	1.17 (1.01–1.35)‡	1.36 (1.04–1.79)§	1.11 (0.93–1.31)
Daytime blood pressure	0.98 (0.83–1.17)	1.07 (0.85–1.34)	1.08 (0.94–1.24)	1.25 (0.97–1.61)	1.03 (0.87–1.21)
Night-time blood pressure	1.14 (1.00–1.30)‡	1.18 (0.98–1.42)†	1.20 (1.08–1.35)§	1.31 (1.06–1.62)‡	1.16 (1.02–1.33)‡

*Relative hazard rates with 95% CI between parentheses reflect the risk associated with a 10 mmHg increase in systolic ambulatory blood pressure. Risk estimates were adjusted for sex, age, previous cardiovascular complications, smoking, residence in western Europe, and the conventional systolic blood pressure at entry.
†$p \leq 0.07$.
‡$p \leq 0.05$.
§$p \leq 0.01$.
¶$p \leq 0.001$.
‖Also adjusted for active treatment.

Active treatment reduced total stroke by 38%, from 20.8 down to 13.0 end-points per 1000 patient–years (CI 9–58%; p = 0.01), all-cause mortality by 39% (CI 16–57%; p = 0.003), cardiovascular mortality by 39% (CI 4–61%; p = 0.03), stroke mortality by 58% (CI 14–80%; p = 0.02), and all fatal and non-fatal cardiovascular end-points by 37% (CI 14–53%; p = 0.004). Treatment of 1000 Chinese patients for 5 years could prevent 55 deaths, 39 strokes, or 59 major cardiovascular end-points.[8]

Outcome in diabetic and non-diabetic patients and other subgroup analyses

Subgroup analyses of the Syst-China results demonstrated that the benefit of antihypertensive treatment was particularly evident in the diabetic Syst-China patients. Of 2394 Syst-China patients, 98 (4.1%) had diabetes. On active treatment, the net placebo-subtracted differences in blood pressure after 2 years were −6.0/−4.7 mmHg in the diabetic patients and −9.3/−3.1 mmHg in the non-diabetic patients. After adjustment for possible confounders, active treatment decreased the relative risk in diabetic and non-diabetic patients as follows: −59% versus −36% for total mortality, −57% versus −33% for cardiovascular mortality, and −74% versus −34% for all cardiovascular end-points. However, because of the small number of diabetic patients, the diabetes-by-treatment interaction terms were not statistically significant. Nevertheless, active treatment reduced the excess cardiovascular mortality and morbidity noticed in the diabetic Syst-China patients to a non-significant level.[36]

For cardiac end-points, the benefit of active treatment tended to be slightly larger in non-smokers (69.2% of all patients).[36] Otherwise, in the Syst-China trial, the benefits of active treatment were not significantly influenced by the entry characteristics of the patients.[36]

Pooled estimates of benefit

The results of the three outcome trials in older patients with isolated systolic hypertension were pooled, using methods described elsewhere.[37,38] Zelen's exact test for homogeneity did not reach statistical significance for any of the end-points considered. Thus, the hypothesis of a common underlying treatment effect across the three studies was not rejected. Overall, compared with placebo, active treatment reduced all-cause mortality by 17% (CI 5–18%; p = 0.008) and cardiovascular mortality by 25% (CI 8–39%; p = 0.005). For the fatal and non-fatal complications combined, these reductions were 32% for all cardiovascular end-points (CI 13–41%; p < 0.001), 37% for stroke (CI 24–38%; p < 0.001), and 25% for myocardial infarction including sudden death (CI 9–39%; p < 0.001).[38]

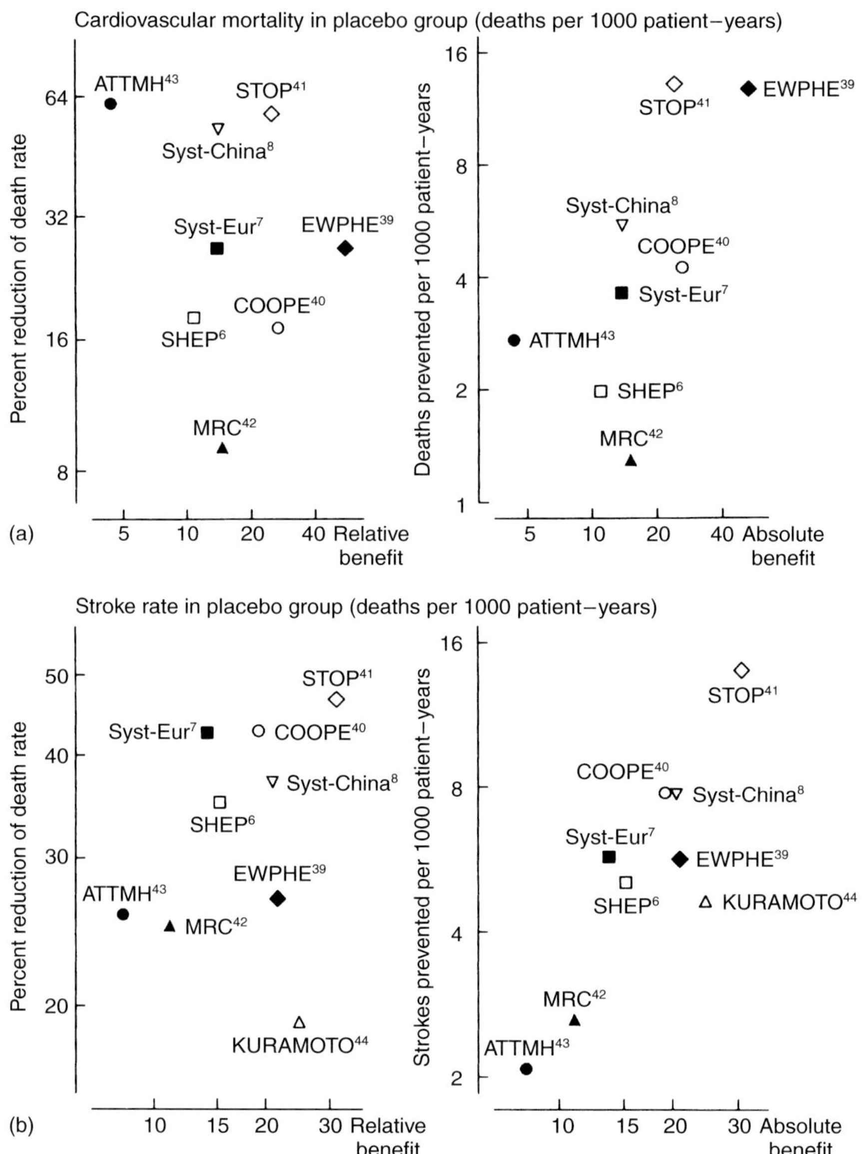

Figure 5.5

Comparison of the relative and absolute benefits of antihypertensive drug treatment with regard to (a) cardiovascular mortality and (b) fatal and non-fatal stroke in older (≥60 years) hypertensive patients enrolled in nine intervention trials.[6–8,39–44]

The benefits of antihypertensive treatment in the trials in isolated systolic hypertension were similar to those in six other trials[39–44] in older patients with combined systolic and diastolic hypertension. Overall, in these six trials, antihypertensive treatment reduced fatal stroke by 33% and cardiovascular mortality by 22%.[37] Whereas the relative benefit of antihypertensive treatment is constant over a wide range of risk, absolute benefit varies widely according to the risk of events experienced in the control group.[45] Among nine intervention trials in the elderly,[6–8,39–44] the number of patients to treat for 1 year to prevent one cardiovascular death or one stroke was at an intermediate level in the three trials[6–8] in isolated systolic hypertension (*Fig. 5.5*).

Comparative results in diabetic patients

Recently, the controversy on the use of calcium channel blockers found new life in a series of articles[46–50] and comments[51] that suggested that calcium channel blockers, including second-generation dihydropyridines such as amlodipine[47] or nisoldipine,[46] might be harmful, particularly in hypertensive patients with diabetes mellitus.

Using the same end-point definitions as in the SHEP trial and similar adjustments for possible confounders, the Syst-Eur investigators compared their outcome results[11] with those observed in SHEP[10] (see *Fig. 5.2*). The validity of these comparisons is sustained by similar net decreases in blood pressure in the active-treatment groups (*Table 5.6*), by the similar rates in the placebo groups of the two trials regardless of the presence of diabetes at randomization (see *Table 5.6*), and by the practically identical relative benefit in terms of outcome in the non-diabetic subpopulations (see *Fig. 5.2*).

The major difference between the two trials was in the outcome of the diabetic patients (see *Fig. 5.2*) in whom three major complications declined two to four times more on dihydropyridine-based treatment[21] than on treatment with chlorthalidone.[10] At the end of the SHEP trial,[6] 44% of the patients randomized to placebo were on active antihypertensive drugs. However, this does not explain the lesser protection conferred by diuretic-initiated treatment in the diabetic patients, because crossing over to active treatment should have affected outcome in diabetic patients as well as non-diabetic patients.

The Syst-Eur findings in diabetic and non-diabetic patients were not only reinforced by the subgroup analysis of the Syst-China trial,[36] but also by recent findings in two other trials.[52,53] Taken together, these observations[21,36,52,53] are in line with the hypothesis that long-acting dihydropyridine calcium channel blockers, rather than low-dose thiazides, may be the drug class of choice to initiate blood pressure lowering in older hypertensive patients who also have diabetes mellitus.[54]

Table 5.6 Results of the SHEP and the Syst-Eur trials in diabetic and non-diabetic patients[21]

	Diabetic patients		Non-diabetic patients	
	SHEP	Syst-Eur	SHEP	Syst-Eur
Number (%)	590 (12.3)	492 (10.5)	4149 (87.7)	4203 (89.5)
Mean blood pressure reduction*				
Systolic (mmHg)	−9.8	−8.6	−12.5	−10.3
Diastolic (mmHg)	−2.2	−3.3	−4.1	−4.6
Risk in placebo group†				
Total mortality	35.6	45.1	21.8	21.6
Cardiovascular end-points	63.0	55.0	36.8	28.9
Stroke	28.8	26.6	15.0	12.3
Coronary events	32.2	23.1	15.2	12.4

*The mean effect of active treatment on blood pressure was corrected for baseline and placebo.
†Rate expressed as events per 1000 patient–years.

The emerging role of pulse pressure as cardiovascular risk factor

The current guidelines for the management of hypertension rest almost completely on the measurement of systolic and diastolic blood pressure, two specific inflection points of the blood pressure wave, which are usually considered in isolation.[31,55] However, blood pressure propagates through the arterial tree as a repetitive continuous wave and is more accurately described as consisting of:

(a) a pulsatile component (pulse pressure), which depends on ventricular ejection, arterial stiffness, and the timing of wave reflections; and
(b) a steady component (mean pressure), the main determinants of which are cardiac output and peripheral vascular resistance.

Several observational studies[57–66] have produced evidence suggesting that, in middle-aged and older people, pulse pressure may be a better predictor of cardiovascular complications than mean pressure. Pulse pressure widens with advancing age,[3] so that the outcome trials in elderly hypertensive patients provided a database that was particularly suitable for exploring the independent roles of pulse pressure and mean pressure as determinants of cardiovascular prognosis. To address this issue with sufficient statistical power, a meta-analysis[67] was performed that included the results of three placebo-controlled trials in elderly hypertensives: the study conducted by the European Working Party on High Blood Pressure in the Elderly (EWPHE)[39,68] and the Syst-Eur[7] and the Syst-China[8] trials.

The risks associated with pulse pressure and mean pressure were adjusted for sex, age, previous cardiovascular complications, smoking, and active treatment.[67] In addition, the relative hazard rates for pulse pressure were also adjusted for mean pressure and vice versa (*Table 5.7*). In each trial, with the single exception of the coronary end-points in the Syst-Eur trial, pulse pressure was associated with a risk ratio greater than unity; the hazard rates were statistically significant for cardiovascular mortality and all cardiovascular end-points in the EWPHE trial, for fatal and non-fatal stroke in the Syst-Eur trial, and for all end-points considered in the analysis in the Syst-China trial. Overall, in Cox regression with stratification for the three trials and with adjustment for the other covariates, a 10 mmHg wider pulse pressure was correlated with an increase in the risk of any end-point by approximately 10–20% (*Table 5.7*).

Mean pressure adjusted for pulse pressure and the same set of possible confounders was not identified as a consistent and significant predictor of risk (see *Table 5.7*). However, without the adjustment for pulse pressure, the hazard rates associated with a 10 mmHg increase in mean pressure were 1.16 (CI 1.03–1.32; $p = 0.02$) for total mortality, 1.17 (CI 0.99–1.38; $p = 0.06$) for cardiovascular mortality, 1.09 (0.98–1.27;

Table 5.7 Adjusted* relative hazard rates associated with a 10 mmHg increase in pulse pressure or in mean blood pressure[67]

Characteristic	EWPHE[39]	Syst-Eur[7]	Syst-China[8]	All§
Pulse pressure¶				
Total mortality	1.09 (0.97–1.23)	1.06 (0.96–1.17)	1.38 (1.23–1.57)‡	1.15 (1.07–1.22)‡
Cardiovascular mortality	1.17 (1.01–1.36)†	1.10 (0.97–1.27)	1.48 (1.27–1.72)‡	1.22 (1.13–1.33)‡
Cardiovascular end-points	1.15 (1.03–1.29)†	1.06 (0.97–1.16)	1.38 (1.24–1.55)‡	1.17 (1.10–1.24)‡
Stroke	1.10 (0.90–1.36)	1.18 (1.03–1.36)†	1.22 (1.04–1.41)†	1.17 (1.07–1.29)‡
Coronary end-points	1.08 (0.90–1.32)	0.97 (0.83–1.12)	1.64 (1.36–2.00)‡	1.13 (1.02–1.24)†
Mean pressure‖				
Total mortality	1.16 (0.94–1.44)	1.02 (0.83–1.23)	0.83 (0.65–1.04)	1.01 (0.90–1.14)
Cardiovascular mortality	1.22 (0.93–1.58)	0.89 (0.68–1.15)	0.72 (0.53–0.99)†	0.97 (0.83–1.13)
Cardiovascular end-points	1.12 (0.90–1.37)	0.93 (0.78–1.12)	0.83 (0.66–1.03)	0.96 (0.86–1.08)
Stroke	1.51 (1.05–2.18)†	0.98 (0.74–1.31)	0.85 (0.63–1.15)	1.06 (0.89–1.27)
Coronary end-points	1.09 (0.77–1.55)	1.05 (0.78–1.41)	0.76 (0.52–1.14)	0.97 (0.80–1.18)

*All hazard rates are presented with 95% CI between parentheses and were adjusted for sex, age, previous cardiovascular complications, smoking and active treatment.
†$p \leq 0.05$.
‡$p \leq 0.001$.
§Stratification of the Cox models accounted for differences between the three trials.
¶Also adjusted for mean pressure.
‖Also adjusted for pulse pressure.

$p = 0.12$) for all cardiovascular end-points, 1.21 (CI 1.00–1.44; $p = 0.05$) for fatal and non-fatal stroke, and 1.08 (CI 0.89–1.32; $p = 0.44$) for fatal and non-fatal coronary end-points.

Conclusions

The pooled results of the three outcome trials in older patients with isolated systolic hypertension prove that antihypertensive drug treatment must be prescribed if, on repeated measurement, systolic blood pressure is $\geq$160 mmHg. The entry diastolic blood pressure level averaged nearly 85 mmHg in the Syst-Eur[7] and Syst-China[8] trials and was as low as 77 mmHg in the SHEP study.[6] These findings negate the hypothesis that vigorously lowering diastolic blood pressure would compromise the coronary circulation and provoke coronary complications rather than prevent them.[69] Furthermore, long-acting dihydropyridines constitute a valid alternative to diuretics and β-blockers[70] in the primary prevention of cardiovascular disorders in elderly hypertensives. In isolated systolic hypertension, calcium channel blockade may be particularly indicated in diabetic patients[11] (see *Fig. 5.2*) and in those at risk of dementia[24] (see *Fig. 5.3*).

In untreated older patients with isolated systolic hypertension, the ambulatory systolic blood pressure, over and above the conventional blood pressure, predicted cardiovascular risk. This was particularly manifest when the ambulatory systolic blood pressure was measured at night or when the 24-hour, daytime or night-time systolic blood pressure exceeded 142 mmHg, 145 mmHg, or 132 mmHg, respectively.[30] The risk conferred by any level of conventional systolic blood pressure at entry in the Syst-Eur trial[30] declined by nearly one-fifth for each 10 mmHg increase in the 'white-coat' effect (conventional blood pressure minus daytime blood pressure). The hypothesis[71] of an inverse association between cardiovascular risk and the blood pressure fall at night was confirmed. The influence of physical and psychoemotional stress may weaken the predictive power of the daytime blood pressure, whereas the greater uniformity resulting from sleeping may help to demonstrate correlations with the night-time blood pressure. The smaller within-subject coefficient of variation for the night-time blood pressure than for the daytime blood pressure was in line with this hypothesis.[30]

In older hypertensive patients pulse pressure—not mean pressure—is the major determinant of cardiovascular risk.[67] The implications of these findings for the management of hypertensive patients should be subject to further investigation in randomized controlled outcome trials, in which the pulsatile component of blood pressure is differently influenced by antihypertensive drug treatment.

References

1. Kannel WB, Gordon T. Evaluation of cardiovascular risk in the elderly: the Framingham study. Bull N Y Acad Med 1978; 54: 573–591.

2. Staessen J, O'Brien E, Atkins N *et al.* The increase in blood pressure with age and body mass index is overestimated by conventional sphygmomanometry. Am J Epidemiol 1992;·136: 450–459.

3. Staessen J, Amery A, Fagard R. Editorial review. Isolated systolic hypertension in the elderly. J Hypertens 1990; 8: 393–405.

4. Buck C, Baker P, Bass M, Donner A. The prognosis of hypertension according to age at onset. Hypertension 1987; 9: 204–208.

5. Thijs L, Fagard R, Lijnen P *et al.* Why is antihypertensive drug therapy needed in elderly patients with systolodiastolic hypertension? J Hypertens 1994; 12 (suppl 6): S25–S34.

6. SHEP Cooperative Research Group. Prevention of stroke by antihypertensive drug treatment in older persons with isolated systolic hypertension. Final results of the Systolic Hypertension in the Elderly Program (SHEP). JAMA 1991; 265: 3255–3264.

7. Staessen JA, Fagard R, Thijs L *et al.* for the Systolic Hypertension in Europe (Syst-Eur) Trial Investigators. Randomised double-blind comparison of placebo and active treatment for older patients with isolated systolic hypertension (erratum published in Lancet 1997; 350: 1636). Lancet 1997; 350: 757–764.

8. Liu L, Wang JG, Gong L *et al.* for the Systolic Hypertension in China (Syst-China) Collaborative Group. Comparison of active treatment and placebo for older patients with isolated systolic hyperten-sion. J Hypertens 1998; 16: 1823–1829.

9. The Systolic Hypertension in the Elderly Program Cooperative Research Group. Implications of the Systolic Hypertension in the Elderly Program. Hypertension 1993; 21: 335–343.

10. Curb JD, Pressel SL, Cutler JA *et al.* for the Systolic Hypertension in the Elderly Cooperative Research Group. Effect of diuretic-based antihypertensive treatment on cardiovascular disease risk in older diabetic patients with isolated systolic hypertension. JAMA 1996; 276: 1886–1892.

11. Tuomilehto J, Rastenyte D, Birkenhäger WH *et al.* for the Systolic Hypertension in Europe (Syst-Eur) Trial Investigators, Staessen JA. Effects of calcium-channel blockade in older patients with diabetes and systolic hypertension. N Engl J Med 1999; 340: 677–684.

12. Amery A, Birkenhäger W, Bulpitt CJ *et al.* Syst-Eur. A multicentre trial on the treatment of isolated systolic hypertension in the elderly: objectives, protocol, and organization. Aging Clin Exp Res 1991; 3: 287–302.

13. Staessen JA, Fagard R, Thijs L *et al.* for the Systolic Hypertension in Europe (Syst-Eur) Trial Investigators. Subgroup and per-protocol analysis of the randomized European trial on isolated systolic hypertension in the elderly. Arch Intern Med 1998; 158: 1681–1691.

14. Fletcher A, Spiegelhalter D, Staessen J *et al.* Implications for trials in progress of publication of positive results. Lancet 1993; 342: 653–657.

15. Kaplan NM. Systolic Hypertension in the Elderly Program (SHEP)

and Swedish Trial in Old Patients With Hypertension (STOP). The promises and the potential problems. Am J Hypertens 1992; 5: 331–334.

16. Ménard J, Day M, Chatellier G, Laragh JH. Some lessons from Systolic Hypertension in the Elderly Program (SHEP). Am J Hypertens 1992; 5: 325–330.

17. Staessen J, Fagard R, Amery A. Isolated systolic hypertension in the elderly: implications of SHEP for clinical practice and for the ongoing trials. J Hum Hypertens 1991; 5: 469–474.

18. Staessen JA, Amery A, Birkenhäger W. Inverse association between baseline pressure and benefit from treatment in isolated systolic hypertension. Hypertension 1994; 23: 269–270.

19. Furberg CD, Psaty BM, Meyer JV. Nifedipine. Dose-related increase in mortality in patients with coronary heart disease. Circulation 1995; 92: 1326–1331.

20. Psaty BM, Heckbert SR, Koepsell TD *et al.* The risk of myocardial infarction associated with antihypertensive drug therapies. JAMA 1995; 274: 620–625.

21. Staessen JA, Thijs L, Fagard RH *et al.* for the Systolic Hypertension in Europe (Syst-Eur) Trial Investigators. Calcium channel blockade and cardiovascular prognosis in the European trial on isolated systolic hypertension. Hypertension 1998; 32: 404–409.

22. Forette F, Amery A, Staessen J *et al.* Is prevention of vascular dementia possible? The Syst-Eur Vascular Dementia Project. Aging Clin Exp Res 1991; 3: 373–382.

23. Seux ML, Thijs L, Forette F *et al.* Correlates of cognitive status of old patients with isolated systolic hypertension: the Syst-Eur Vascular Dementia Project. J Hypertens 1998; 16: 963–969.

24. Forette F, Seux ML, Staessen JA *et al.* on behalf of the Syst-Eur Investigators. Prevention of dementia in randomised double-blind placebo-controlled Systolic Hypertension in Europe (Syst-Eur) trial. Lancet 1998; 352: 1347–1351.

25. Folstein MF, Folstein SE, McHugh PR. 'Mini-Mental State'. A practical method for grading the cognitive state of patients for the clinician. J Psychiat Res 1975; 12: 189–198.

26. Diagnostic and Statistical Manual of Mental Disorders III. Washington, DC USA: American Psychiatric Association, 1987.

27. Staessen JA, Thijs L, Birkenhäger WH *et al.* on behalf of the Syst-Eur Investigators. Update on the Systolic Hypertension in Europe (Syst-Eur) Trial. Hypertension 1999; 33: 1476–1477.

28. Staessen J, Amery A, Clement D *et al.* Twenty-four hour blood pressure monitoring in the Syst-Eur trial. Aging Clin Exp Res 1992; 4: 85–91.

29. Emelianov D, Thijs L, Staessen JA *et al.* on behalf of the Syst-Eur Investigators. Conventional and ambulatory blood pressure measurement in older patients with isolated systolic hypertension: baseline observations in the Syst-Eur trial. Blood Press Monit 1998; 3: 173–180.

30. Staessen JA, Thijs L, Fagard R for the Systolic Hypertension in Europe (Syst-Eur) Trial Investigators. Predicting cardiovascular risk using conventional vs ambulatory blood pressure in older patients with systolic hypertension. JAMA 1999; 286: 539–546.

31. The Joint National Committee on Prevention Detection Evaluation and Treatment of High Blood Pressure. The sixth report of the Joint National Committee on

Prevention, Detection, Evaluation, and Treatment of High Blood Pressure (JNC VI). Arch Intern Med 1997; 157: 2413–2446.

32. Staessen JA, O'Brien ET, Amery AK. Ambulatory blood pressure in normotensive and hypertensive subjects: results from an international database. J Hypertens 1994; 12 (suppl 7): S1–S12.

33. Fagard R, Brguljan J, Thijs L, Staessen J. Prediction of the actual awake and asleep blood pressures by various methods of 24 h pressure analysis. J Hypertens 1996; 14: 557–563.

34. Collaborative Group Coordinating Center. Systolic hypertension in the elderly: Chinese trial (Syst-China)—Interim report. Chin J Cardiol 1992; 20: 270–275.

35. Wang J, Liu G, Wang X *et al.* on behalf of the Syst-China Investigators. Long-term blood pressure control in older Chinese patients with isolated systolic hypertension: a progress report on the Syst-China trial. J Hum Hypertens 1996; 10: 735–742.

36. Wang JG, Staessen JA, Gong L, Liu L for the Systolic Hypertension in China Investigator. Subgroup analysis of the placebo-controlled Chinese trial on isolated systolic hypertension in the elderly. Arch Intern Med 2000; in press.

37. Thijs L, Fagard R, Lijnen P *et al.* A meta-analysis of outcome trials in elderly hypertensives. J Hypertens 1992; 10: 1103–1109.

38. Staessen JA, Wang JG. Benefit of antihypertensive drug treatment in older patients with isolated systolic hypertension. Eur Heart J Suppl 1999; 1 (suppl P): P3–P8

39. Amery A, Birkenhäger W, Brixko P *et al.* Mortality and morbidity results from the European Working Party on High Blood Pressure in the Elderly trial. Lancet 1985; i: 1349–1354.

40. Coope J, Warrender TS. Randomised trial of treatment of hypertension in elderly patients in primary care. BMJ 1986; 293: 1145–1151.

41. Dahlöf B, Lindholm LH, Hansson L *et al.* Morbidity and mortality in the Swedish Trial in Old Patients with Hypertension (STOP-Hypertension). Lancet 1991; 338: 1281–1285.

42. MRC Working Party. Medical Research Council trial of treatment of hypertension in older adults: principal results. BMJ 1992; 304: 405–412.

43. Management Committee. Treatment of mild hypertension in the elderly. A study initiated and administered by the National Heart Foundation of Australia. Med J Aust 1981; 2: 398–402.

44. Kuramoto K, Matsushita S, Kuwajima I, Murakami M. Prospective study on the treatment of mild hypertension in the aged. Jpn Heart J 1981; 22: 75–85.

45. Lever AF, Ramsay LE. Treatment of hypertension in the elderly (editorial review). J Hypertens 1995; 13: 571–579.

46. Estacio RO, Jeffers BW, Hiatt WR *et al.* The effect of nisoldipine as compared with enalapril on cardiovascular outcomes in patients with non-insulin-dependent diabetes and hypertension. N Engl J Med 1998; 338: 645–652.

47. Tatti P, Pahor M, Byington RB *et al.* Outcome results of the Fosinopril versus Amlodipine Cardiovascular Events Randomized Trial (FACET) in patients with hypertension and NIDDM. Diabetes Care 1998; 21: 597–603.

48. Alderman M, Madhavan S, Cohen H. Calcium antagonists and cardiovascular events in patients with hypertension and diabetes. Lancet 1998; 351: 216–217.

49. Byington RP, Craven TE, Furberg

CD, Pahor M. Isradipine, raised glycosylated haemoglobin, and risk of cardiovascular events. Lancet 1998; 350: 1075–1076.

50. Pahor M, Kritchevsky SB, Zuccala G, Guralnik JM. Diabetes and risk of adverse events with calcium antagonists. Diabetes Care 1998; 21: 193–194.

51. Pahor M, Psaty BM, Furberg CD. Treatment of hypertensive patients with diabetes. Lancet 1998; 351: 689–690.

52. Cutler JA. Calcium-channel blockers for hypertension: uncertainty continues. N Engl J Med 1998; 338: 679–681.

53. Hansson L, Zanchetti A, Carruthers SG *et al.* for the HOT Study Group. Effects of intensive blood pressure lowering and low-dose aspirin in patients with hypertension: principal results of the Hypertension Optimal Treatment (HOT) randomised trial. Lancet 1998; 351: 1755–1762.

54. Birkenhäger WH, Staessen JA. Treatment of diabetic patients with hypertension. Curr Hypertens Rep 1999; 3: 225–231.

55. Guidelines Subcommittee. 1999 World Health Organization–International Society of Hypertension guidelines for the management of hypertension. J Hypertens 1999; 17: 151–183.

56. Nichols WW, O'Rourke MF. Properties of the arterial wall: theory. In: Nichols WW, O'Rourke MF, eds. McDonald's Blood Flow in Arteries: Theoretical, Experimental and Clinical Principles. London, UK: Edward Arnold, 1998, 54–72.

57. Darné B, Girerd X, Safar M *et al.* Pulsatile versus steady component of blood pressure: a cross-sectional analysis and a prospective analysis on cardiovascular mortality. Hypertension 1989; 13: 392–400.

58. Rutan GH, Kuller LH, Neaton JD *et al.* Mortality associated with diastolic hypertension and isolated systolic hypertension among men screened for the Multiple Risk Factor Intervention Trial. Circulation 1988; 77: 504–514.

59. Wilking SVB, Belanger AI, Kannel WB *et al.* Determinants of isolated systolic hypertension. JAMA 1988; 260: 3451–3455.

60. Millar JA, Lever AF. Pulse pressure predicts coronary but not cerebrovascular events in placebo-treated male subjects of the MRC trial. J Hypertens 1996; 14 (suppl 1): S194.

61. Benetos A, Safar M, Rudnichi A *et al.* Pulse pressure. A predictor of long-term cardiovascular mortality in a French male population. Hypertension 1997; 30: 1410–1415.

62. Madhavan S, Ooi WL, Cohen H, Alderman MH. Relation of pulse pressure and blood pressure reduction to the incidence of myocardial infarction. Hypertension 1994; 23: 395–401.

63. Fang J, Madhavan S, Cohen H, Alderman MH. Measures of blood pressure and myocardial infarction in treated hypertensive patients. J Hypertens 1995; 13: 413–419.

64. Mitchel GF, Moyé LA, Braunwald E *et al.* for the SAVE Investigators. Sphygmomanometrically determined pulse pressure is a powerful independent predictor of recurrent events after myocardial infarction in patients with impaired left ventricular function. Circulation 1997; 96: 4254–4260.

65. Franklin SS, Gustin WIV, Wong ND *et al.* Hemodynamic patterns of age-related changes in blood pressure. The Framingham Heart Study. Circulation 1997; 96: 308–315.

66. Neaton JD, Wentworth D for the

Multiple Risk Factor Intervention Trial Research Group. Serum cholesterol, blood pressure, cigarette smoking, and death from coronary heart disease. Overall findings and differences by age for 316,099 white men. Arch Intern Med 1992; 152: 56–64.

67. Blacher J, Staessen JA, Girerd X *et al.* Pulse pressure—not mean pressure—determines cardiovascular risk in older hypertensive patients. Arch Intern Med 2000; in press.

68. Amery A, Birkenhäger W, Brixko P *et al.* Efficacy of antihypertensive drug treatment according to age, sex, blood pressure, and previous cardiovascular disease in patients over the age of 60. Lancet 1986; ii: 589–592.

69. Cruickshank JM, Thorp JM, Zacharias FJ. Benefits and potential harm of lowering high blood pressure. Lancet 1987; i: 581–583.

70. Staessen JA, Wang JG, Birkenhäger WH, Fagard R. Treatment with beta-blockers for the primary prevention of the cardiovascular complications of hypertension. Eur Heart J 1999; 20: 11–25.

71. O'Brien E, Sheridan J, O'Malley K. Dippers and non-dippers. Lancet 1988; ii: 397.

6

The calcium antagonist controversy: has it been settled?

Franz H Messerli and Ehud Grossman

Introduction

Calcium antagonists are widely used as antihypertensive agents, and their use has increased dramatically over the past decade.[1] Their wide appeal can be attributed to several features including their antihypertensive efficacy, metabolic neutrality, and tolerability. If one accepts the surrogate end-point of lowering blood pressure as the goal of antihypertensive treatment, calcium antagonists could be considered to be near-ideal agents.

However, as with most drug classes, longitudinal studies documenting efficacy in preventing stroke, myocardial infarction, congestive heart failure, or death are sparse. Recent reports have shown that hypertensive patients treated with short-acting calcium antagonists are at increased risk of myocardial infarction and have a higher mortality rate than patients treated with other antihypertensive drugs.[2–5]

These findings were widely publicized by the news media and caused anxiety and even panic among patients, some of whom discontinued their antihypertensive drugs altogether; physicians whose offices were inundated by phone calls were frustrated because of the complete lack of information available. Although this panic was unnecessary and unfortunate, the principal question raised by these studies, however imperfect—whether calcium antagonists as individual agents or as a class promote adverse cardiovascular events—deserves further consideration.

Recently, a few retrospective studies have been published that attest to the safety of calcium antagonists.[6–8] Several prospective studies have reported that calcium antagonists exert a beneficial effect on morbidity and mortality in patients with congestive heart failure resulting from dilated cardiomyopathy, in post-myocardial infarction patients, and in hypertensive patients.[9–13]

The evidence for and against calcium antagonists should be weighed solely on its scientific merits. Therefore, several points need to be clarified before one can reach a conclusion.

Calcium antagonists are a heterogeneous class of drug

Not all calcium antagonists are created equal; therefore, one can not assume that all calcium antagonists are equally dangerous or equally beneficial. Psaty *et al.*,[3] in a retrospective case control study, showed a significant increase in the relative risk for myocardial infarction only with verapamil and diltiazem but not with nifedipine. In contrast, Pahor *et al.*,[5] in a retrospective cohort study of elderly patients, showed that only nifedipine, and not verapamil or diltiazem, was associated with increased mortality risk.

Thus, even studies that implicate calcium antagonists as a class for promoting cardiovascular events attest, at a closer look, to the heterogeneity of this effect. Calcium antagonists differ in their molecular structure, their sites and modes of action on the slow calcium channel, and their effects on various other cardiovascular function. For example, verapamil is less vasoselective, has more negative inotropic effects and elicits less activation of both the autonomic nervous system and the renin–angiotensin cascade than dihydropyridine calcium antagonists. Verapamil, therefore, may be more adequate for hypertensive patients with ischemic heart disease, particularly after myocardial infarction.[9,10] Conversely, amlodipine, which has little negative inotropic effect, may be beneficial in selected patients with congestive heart failure.[11]

Effects are dose dependent (*Sola dosis facit venenum*)

The increased risk of cardiovascular events or mortality that occurred with short-acting calcium antagonists was associated only with medium and large doses of these agents.[3,4] Neither the case–control study[3] nor the meta-analysis[4] showed a significant increase in the risk ratio with the low-dose calcium antagonists. Similarly, the risk ratio for mortality was significantly increased only in those who used a high dose of nifedipine in the cohort study.[5] In contrast, Reicher-Reiss *et al.*[14] demonstrated no increase in morbidity and mortality risk in patients with an acute myocardial infarction who were treated for 1 year with short-acting nifedipine (10 mg q8h). In this study, the 5-year mortality risk of patients who were randomized to nifedipine was exactly the same as that of those who were randomized to placebo. These findings are similar to those of a case–control study with thiazide diuretics, in which a higher dose of thiazide was associated with a 3.5-fold increase in the risk of cardiac arrest compared with the lower dose.[15] It may not be the drug *per se* but the dose that determines the risk of cardiovascular events.

Long-acting versus short-acting calcium antagonists

All retrospective studies that have purported to show increased risk with calcium antagonists used the short-acting agents. Short-acting calcium antagonists rapidly attain a plasma concentration that is prone to reduce blood pressure markedly and to stimulate the sympathetic nervous system. Although this stimulation is more marked with the first dose, it persists even with prolonged therapy of short-acting calcium antagonists (*Fig. 6.1*).[16] A precipitous fall in blood pressure in association with sympathetic stimulation may decrease coronary blood flow and increase oxygen demand and thereby increase rate of myocardial ischemia, particularly in patients with underlying ischemic heart disease. Indeed, with sublingual nifedipine, the use of which has been widespread for treatment of what were perceived as hypertensive emergencies, serious and even fatal adverse effects have been reported.[17] These complications are not unique to sublingual nifedipine and can be observed with any other powerful vasodilator as well. However, given that the benefits of lowering arterial pressure by sublingual nifedipine in hypertensive emergencies has never been established, even one fatality must be considered too many.

Another factor to be considered in this context is the activity of the sympathetic nervous system. Increased sympathetic activity has been shown to represent one of the non-pressure-related coronary risk factors

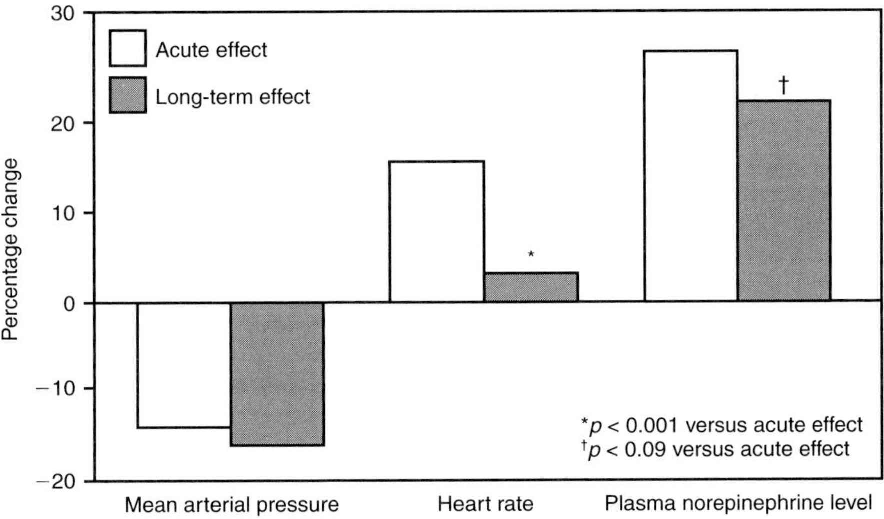

Figure 6.1

Acute and long-term effects of short-acting calcium antagonists.

in hypertension. It may directly and indirectly cause the development or maintenance of left ventricular hypertrophy and atherosclerosis, and it may potentiate cardiac arrhythmias and sudden death.[18] Recent studies have shown that variability in blood pressure, independent of the absolute level, correlates with end-organ damage in hypertensive patients.[19,20] Short-acting drugs do not achieve smooth blood pressure control, and their use is associated with major fluctuations in blood pressure. Thus, the use of short-acting drugs may fail to attenuate end-organ damage even though they decrease blood pressure control. The theoretical disadvantages of short-acting calcium antagonists do not apply to long-acting formulations that achieve a more gradual and sustained antihypertensive effect and therefore avoid activating the sympathetic nervous system.

For example, distinct differences are observed between short-acting and long-acting nifedipine. Whereas short-acting nifedipine produces an increase in heart rate and circulating catecholamines, with the once-daily formulation, both heart rate and circulating catecholamine levels remain unchanged (*Fig. 6.2*). Alderman *et al.*[21] recently documented a 4–8 fold lower relative risk ratio of morbidity and mortality in patients taking a long-acting calcium antagonist compared with those taking a short-acting one. A prospective study, the Shanghai Trial of Nifedipine in the Elderly (STONE),[12] which compared long-acting nifedipine with placebo in a group of 1632 elderly hypertensive patients, showed a significant reduction of 59% for all events and of 62% for combined cardiovascular events in the active treatment arm. The Systolic Hypertension in Europe (Syst-Eur) study[22] has provided iron-clad data attesting to the safety and efficacy of calcium antagonists. In this study, more than 4000 elderly patients with isolated systolic hypertension were randomly assigned to a calcium antagonist (nitrendipine) or placebo.[22] The study was terminated early because of a 42% reduction in stroke rate in the calcium antagonist arm. The study also revealed highly significant reductions in the rates of cardiac end-points and cardiovascular events.

Is the diabetic hypertensive patient different?

A comparison of Syst-Eur with the Systolic Hypertension in the Elderly Program (SHEP) study[23] has shown that there was no difference in the reduction of morbidity and mortality between a diuretic and a calcium blocker in the subjects without diabetes mellitus; a significantly greater benefit was achieved with a calcium antagonist in the hypertensive patients with diabetes. In fact, in the 10% of patients in Syst-Eur who had diabetes, the benefits of antihypertensive therapy with a calcium antagonist strategy were much more pronounced than in the non-diabetic population.[24]

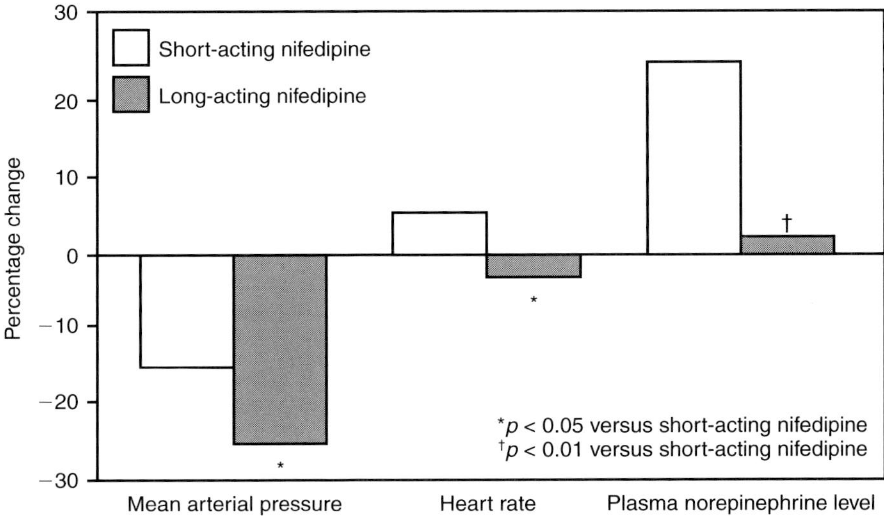

Figure 6.2

Effects of short- and long-acting nifedipine.

These data, attesting to benefits of long-acting dihydropyridine calcium antagonists in hypertensive patients with diabetes, are not necessarily in conflict with those of the Appropriate Blood Pressure Control in Diabetes (ABCD) study,[25] which found no difference, in a similar population, between an angiotensin converting enzyme inhibitor and the long-acting dihydropyridine calcium antagonist in primary outcome (renal function), although admittedly in this study more patients taking the calcium antagonists had myocardial infarction.

It must be emphasized, however, that the ABCD trial was designed to study changes in creatinine clearance, and myocardial infarction was only a secondary end-point. Unfortunately, the treatment status and the doses of study medication being used at the time of infarction were not reported. Moreover, more patients in the ACE inhibitor arm received diuretics (119 versus 93, $p < 0.02$) and β-blockers (95 versus 89, $p < 0.04$). In addition, more patients in the nisoldipine group than in the enalapril group stopped taking the study medication. For all these reasons, overall cardiovascular outcome may have been better in the enalapril than in the nisoldipine group.

Since a placebo arm was lacking in that study, the absolute reduction in rates of myocardial infarction could not be compared between the two treatment groups. At the very most, one may conclude from this study that perhaps ACE inhibitors have a more favorable effect in the hypertensive patient with diabetes than calcium antagonists do, but not that calcium antagonists are harmful.

A recent study of hypertensive patients with diabetes and left ventricular hypertrophy is interesting in this regard.[26] In a 48-week follow-up, nitrendipine decreased arterial pressure and, in parallel, decreased left ventricular mass. In contrast, despite a similar decrease in arterial pressure, enalapril did not decrease left ventricular mass. This difference is astonishing because ACE inhibitors have been believed to be the most powerful drug class for decreasing left ventricular hypertrophy. The fact that in the hypertensive patient with diabetes the activity of the renin–angiotensin–aldosterone cascade is often low (hyporeninemic hypoaldosteronism) could, to some extent, account for the relative inefficacy of the ACE inhibitor on left ventricular mass when compared with the calcium antagonist.

Do calcium antagonists increase the risk of malignancy?

Cardiovascular disorders such as hypertension, hyperlipidemia, and arrhythmias often require treatment for years and even decades. Since the morbidity and mortality of these disorders (particularly when mild) are relatively low, the benefits from treatment are comparatively small. Thus, the British Medical Research Council study[27] allows us to calculate that almost 1000 patients need to be exposed to antihypertensive therapy with a diuretic for 1 year to prevent a single stroke. Diuretic drugs are comparatively powerful drugs in preventing stroke and benefits are easy to demonstrate. In contrast, the effects of β-blockers on strokes and the benefits of β-blockers and diuretics on coronary artery disease are considerably smaller. This means that numerous patients will be exposed to the adverse effects and cost of these drugs without harvesting any real benefit. Given this scenario of small benefits and long-term exposure, any potential risk of malignancy associated with drugs to treat chronic cardiovascular disorders has to be taken very seriously.

Chemical agents can increase the risk of malignancy either by being directly carcinogenic or by impeding the immune response or apoptosis, or both. Direct carcinogenicity usually requires many years and even decades of exposure and is specific for certain malignancies only. In contrast, the effects of these immunosuppressive agents on apoptosis can manifest themselves within a much shorter period and affect a much larger spectrum of malignancies. It is apoptosis that is purported to be affected by calcium antagonists. In this regard, several studies provide some reassurance. In a cohort of more than 11,000 patients, half of whom were receiving a calcium antagonist, Braun et al.[28] observed no increase in malignancy. Notably, most patients were receiving the short-

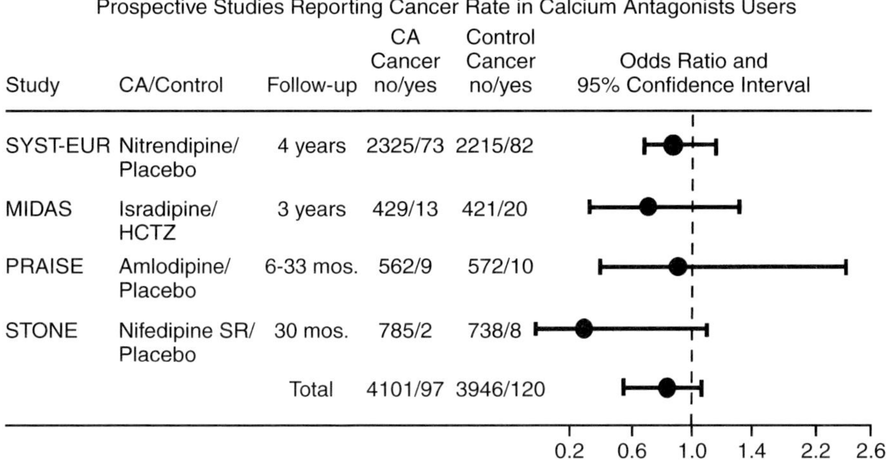

Prospective Studies Reporting Cancer Rate in Calcium Antagonists Users

Study	CA/Control	Follow-up	CA Cancer no/yes	Control Cancer no/yes	Odds Ratio and 95% Confidence Interval
SYST-EUR	Nitrendipine/ Placebo	4 years	2325/73	2215/82	
MIDAS	Isradipine/ HCTZ	3 years	429/13	421/20	
PRAISE	Amlodipine/ Placebo	6-33 mos.	562/9	572/10	
STONE	Nifedipine SR/ Placebo	30 mos.	785/2	738/8	
		Total	4101/97	3946/120	

Figure 6.3

Prospective studies reporting cancer rate in calcium antagonists users. SYST-EUR = Systolic Hypertension in Europe; MIDAS = Multicenter Isradipine Diurectic Atherosclerosis Study; PRAISE = Prospective Randomized Amlodipine Survival Evaluation Study; STONE = Shanghai Trial of Nifedipine in the Elderly. HCTZ = hydrochlorothiazide.

acting forms of nifedipine, diltiazem, and verapamil—the same drugs that in much smaller studies were implicated in carcinogenicity. Several other studies from powerful databases also refute the hypothesis that calcium antagonists increase the risk of nalignancies. In more than 4000 patients in the West of Scotland Cancer Surveillance Unit,[29] a retrospective analysis showed no increased malignancy risk. Similarly, a Danish cohort study[30] of more than 17,000 patients showed no excess malignancy risk in those taking a calcium antagonist. In all four prospective randomized trials assessing morbidity and mortality, the malignancy risk was lower in patients receiving calcium antagonists than in those receiving either placebo or diuretics (*Fig. 6.3*).[11,12,22,31] Perhaps the most powerful data refuting the hypothesis that calcium antagonists alter apoptosis come from the Mayo Clinic. In 621 post-transplant patients with immunosuppression by cyclosporin, Texor *et al.*[32] found no excess malignancy risk in those receiving calcium antagonists (despite comparable immunosuppression) compared with those who were not.

The authors have recently conducted a meta-analysis of all (nine) published observational studies. These studies involve 13,285 calcium antagonist users and 19,625 non-users, who were followed for several years. A similar risk for malignancy among users and non-users was found. In addition, in an observational study of 17,911 patients in Denmark, followed for 3 years, calcium antagonist users had a similar incidence of malignancy as expected by age- and sex-matched populations.

Thus, it is extremely unlikely that calcium antagonists increase the risk of malignancy by affecting either apoptosis or immunosuppression. Although we can be reassured to a great extent by existing data, we shall have to continue to be vigilant with regard to the carcinogenicity of all drugs that are used to treat cardiovascular disorders for years and decades.

Conclusion

Considering the data available in 1999, the authors believe that short-acting calcium antagonists should no longer be used for treatment of hypertension. The practice of using oral or sublingual nifedipine in a hypertensive emergency or pseudoemergency should be abandoned because it can lead to syncope, myocardial infarction, stroke, and death.[17] However, the use of a low dose of the long-acting formulations appears to be safe and promising in patients with essential hypertension.

Despite the availability of many antihypertensive drugs, only 26% of US patients with hypertension have their condition well controlled (blood pressure less than 140/90 mmHg).[33] Therefore, long-acting calcium antagonists should continue to be a cornerstone in the treatment strategy. In hypertensive patients with diabetes, lowering blood pressure with calcium antagonists is clearly beneficial and may have a particular advantage in patients with left ventricular hypertrophy.

The calcium antagonist controversy was helpful in alerting physicians to the fact that hypertension remains a surrogate end-point and that not all drugs that decrease blood pressure will, *paribus passu*, reduce morbidity and mortality. A prime example of failure of the so-called surrogate end-point concept is provided by the authors' recent meta-analysis in hypertension in the elderly. Although β-blockers did lower blood pressure, they consistently failed to decrease the rate of myocardial infarction and cardiovascular and all-cause mortality.[34] This means that numerous elderly hypertensive patients are exposed to adverse effects, inconvenience, and cost of β-blockers without harvesting any benefits.

The excessive news media coverage of the calcium blocker controversy was inappropriate and led to panic and confusion among patients and frustration among physicians. Perhaps we should remember the first rule of treatment set forth by Sir George Pickering: 'Never frighten your patients'.[35]

References

1. Leader SG, Mallick R, Briggs NC. Myocardial infarction in newly diagnosed hypertensive Medicaid patients free of coronary heart disease and treated with calcium channel blockers. Am J Med 1997; 102: 150–157.

2. Borhani NO, Mercuri M, Borhani PA, Buckalew VM *et al.* Final outcome results of the Multicenter Isradipine Diuretic Atherosclerosis Study (MIDAS). A randomized controlled trial. JAMA 1996; 276: 785–791.

3. Psaty BM, Heckbert SR, Koepsell TD *et al.* The risk of myocardial infarction associated with antihypertensive drug therapies. JAMA 1995; 274: 620–625.

4. Furberg CD, Psaty BM, Meyer JV. Nifedipine: dose-related increase in mortality in patient with coronary heart disease. Circulation 1995; 92: 1326–1331.

5. Pahor M, Guralnik JM, Corti MC *et al.* Long-term survival and use of antihypertensive medications in older persons. J Am Geriatr Soc 1995; 43: 1191–1197.

6. Braun S, Boyko V, Behar S *et al.* Calcium antagonists and mortality in patients with coronary artery disease: a cohort study of 11,575 patients. J Am Coll Cardiol 1996; 28: 7–11.

7. Aursnes I, Litleskare I, Froyland H, Abdelnoor M. Association between various drugs used for hypertension and risk of acute myocardial infarction. Blood Pressure 1995; 4: 157–163.

8. Jick H, Derby LE, Gurewich V, Vasilakis C. The risk of myocardial infarction associated with antihypertensive drug treatment in persons with uncomplicated essential hypertension. Pharmacotherapy 1996; 16: 321–326.

9. Danish Study Group on Verapamil in Myocardial Infarction. Effect of verapamil on mortality and major events after acute myocardial infarction (The Danish Verapamil Infarction Trial-II-DAVIT II). Am J Cardiol 1990; 66: 779–785.

10. Multicenter Diltiazem Postinfarction Trial Research Group. The effect of diltiazem on mortality and reinfarction after myocardial infarction. N Engl J Med 1988; 319: 385–392.

11. Packer M, O'Connor CM, Ghali JK *et al.* for the Prospective Randomized Amlodipine Survival Evaluation Study Group (PRAISE). Effect of amlodipine on morbidity and mortality in severe chronic heart failure. N Engl J Med 1996; 335: 1107–1114.

12. Gong L, Zhan W, Zhu Y *et al.* Shanghai Trial of Nifedipine in the Elderly (STONE). J Hypertens 1996; 14: 1237–1245.

13. The DEFIANT-II Research Group. Doppler flow and echocardiography in functional cardiac insufficiency: Assessment of nisoldipine therapy. Results of the DEFIANT-II Study. Eur Heart J 1997; 18: 31–40.

14. Reicher-Reiss H, Behar S, Boyko V *et al.* Long-term mortality follow-up of hospital survivors of a myocardial infarction randomized to nifedipine in the SPRINT study. Secondary Prevention Reinfarction Israeli Nifedipine Trial. Cardiovasc Drugs Ther 1998; 12: 171–176.

15. Siscovick DS, Raghunathan TE, Psaty BM *et al.* Diuretic therapy for hypertension and the risk of primary cardiac arrest. N Engl J Med 1994; 330: 1852–1857.

16. Grossman E, Messerli FH. Effect of calcium antagonists on plasma, norepinephrine levels, heart rate, and blood pressure. Am J Cardiol 1997; 80: 1453–1458.

17. Grossman E, Messerli EH, Grodzicki T, Kowey P. Should a moratorium be placed on nifedipine capsules in hypertensive emergencies and pseudoemergencies? JAMA 1996; 276: 1328–1331.

18. Ruzicka M, Leenen FH. Relevance of 24 H blood pressure profile and sympathetic activity for outcome on short- versus long-acting 1,4-dihydropyridines. Am J Hypertens 1996; 9: 86–94.

19. Parati G, Pomidossi G, Albini F, Malaspina D, Mancia G. Relationship of 24-hour blood pressure mean and variability to severity of target-organ damage in hypertension. J Hypertens 1987; 5: 93–98.

20. Frattola A, Parati G, Cuspidi C *et al.* Prognostic value of 24-hour blood pressure variability. J Hypertens 1993; 11: 1133–1137.

21. Alderman MH, Cohen HW, Roqué R, Madhavan S. The risk of cardiovascular morbidity and mortality associated with calcium channel blockers in antihypertensive therapy. Lancet 1999; in press.

22. Staessen JA, Fagard R, Thijs L *et al.* Randomised double-blind comparison of placebo and active treatment for older patients with isolated systolic hypertension. The Systolic Hypertension in Europe (Syst-Eur) Trial Investigators. Lancet 1997; 350: 757–764.

23. SHEP Cooperative Research Group. Prevention of stroke by antihypertensive drug treatment in older persons with isolated systolic hypertension: final results of the Systolic Hypertension in the Elderly Program (SHEP). JAMA 1991; 265: 3255–3264.

24. Tuomilehto J, Rastenyte D, Birkenhäger WH *et al.* for the Systolic Hypertension in Europe (Syst-Eur) Trial Investigators. Cardiovascular prognosis in older diabetic and nondiabetic patients treated or untreated for isolated systolic hypertension. N Engl J Med 1999; 340: 677–684.

25. Estacio RO, Jeffers BW, Hiatt WR *et al.* The effect of nisoldipine as compared with enalapril on cardiovascular outcomes in patients with non-insulin-dependent diabetes and hypertension. N Engl J Med 1998; 338: 645–652.

26. Gerritsen TA, Bak AAA, Stolk RP *et al.* Effects of nitrendipine and enalapril on left ventricular mass in patients with non-insulin-dependent diabetes mellitus and hypertension. J Hypertens 1998; 16: 689–696.

27. MRC Working Party. Medical Research Council trial of treatment of hypertension in older adults: principal results. BMJ 1985; 291: 97–104.

28. Braun S, Boyko V, Behar S *et al.* Calcium channel blocking agents and risk of cancer in patients with coronary heart disease. Benzafibrate Infarction Prevention (BIP) Study Research Group. J Am Coll Cardiol 1998; 31: 804–808.

29. Hole DJ, Gillis CR, McCallum IR *et al.* Cancer risk of hypertensive patients taking calcium antagonists. J Hypertens 1998; 16: 119–124.

30. Olsen JH Sørensen HT, Frijs S *et al.* Cancer risk in users of calcium channel blockers. Hypertension 1997; 29: 1091–1094.

31. Borhani NO, Mercuri M, Borhani PA *et al.* Final outcome results of the Multicenter Isradipine Diuretic Atherosclerosis Study (MIDAS). A randomized controlled trial. JAMA 1996; 276: 785–791.

32. Textor SC, Taler SJ, Canzanello VJ *et al.* Cancer after liver transplantation (TX): excess risk associated with calcium channel blocker administration (abstract). Am J Hypertens 1997; 10: 199A.

33. Burt VL, Whelton P, Roccella EJ *et al*. Prevalence of hypertension in the US adult population. Results from the Third National Health and Nutrition Examination Survey, 1988–1991. Hypertension 1995; 25: 305–313.

34. Messerli FH, Grossman E, Goldbourt U. Are β-blockers efficacious as first-line therapy for hypertension in the elderly? A systematic review. JAMA 1998; 279: 1903–1907.

35. Pickering GA. Part I: Hypertension. Definitions, natural histories, and consequences. In: Laragh JH, Brenner BM, eds. Hypertension: Pathophysiology, Diagnosis, and Management, vol. 1, 2nd edn. New York: Raven Press, 1995; 3–21.

7
Angiotensin II receptor blockers: will they replace or add to angiotensin converting enzyme inhibitors?

Michel Burnier and Hans R Brunner

Introduction

In the past 15 years, blockade of the renin–angiotensin system with angiotensin converting enzyme (ACE) inhibitors has become an effective and widely used approach to treat hypertension and congestive heart failure as well as a standard therapeutic intervention for the prevention of diabetic and non-diabetic nephropathies. Despite their recognized clinical efficacy, ACE inhibitors have some side effects, such as cough and angioedema, which occasionally limit their prescription and might explain a relative under-use in some indications such as heart failure.[1]

To overcome the drawbacks of ACE inhibition, a great effort has been put into the development of new compounds that block the renin–angiotensin system more specifically.[2] Today, at least six new specific, non-peptide, orally active angiotensin II receptor antagonists (losartan, valsartan, irbesartan, candesartan, telmisartan, and eprosartan) have received approval in the USA from the Food and Drug Administration for the treatment of hypertension and have appeared on the market in many countries. The prescription of these antagonists has experienced a very rapid growth and today, although several large clinical trials are still ongoing with angiotensin II receptor antagonists, one can reasonably ask the question: are angiotensin II receptor blockers going to replace ACE inhibitors or will they be used in combination with ACE inhibitors? This chapter discusses the data that are available so far that may indicate an answer to this question.

The renin–angiotensin system

The renin–angiotensin system starts with the cleavage of angiotensinogen by renin to produce angiotensin I (*Fig. 7.1*). Angiotensin I is then

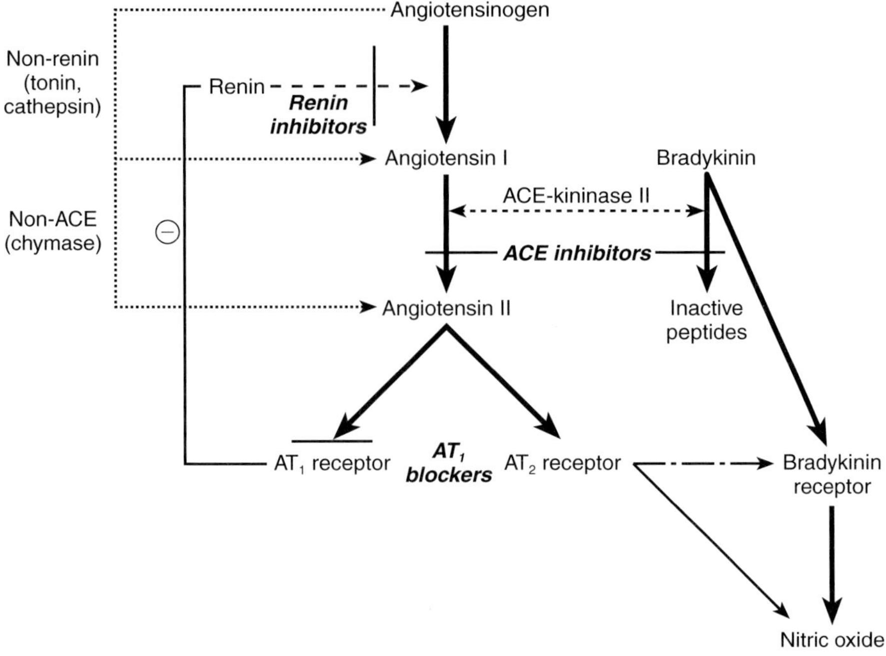

Figure 7.1

The renin–angiotensin system.

converted by ACE (located on endothelial cells in the lungs and in many other vascular beds and on membranes of various cells) to generate angiotensin II. ACE is not a specific enzyme, since it uses bradykinin as a substrate in addition to angiotensin I. In some tissues, angiotensin II may be formed by other enzymatic pathways including, for example, the heart chymase.[3]

Circulating angiotensin II exerts powerful effects on several vascular beds and organ tissues. The multiple effects of angiotensin II (*Table 7.1*) are mediated by the stimulation of specific angiotensin receptors. The development of angiotensin II blockers has led to the recognition and characterization of two main angiotensin receptor subtypes, AT_1 and AT_2. These receptors display a heterogeneous distribution in tissues. So far, all the physiologically significant effects of angiotensin II have been attributed to the stimulation of the AT_1 receptor subtype. AT_2 receptors appear to be important in the fetus and possibly for cell growth. During recent years, several new AT_2-mediated actions of angiotensin II have been proposed (see *Table 7.1*). Thus, there appear to be experimental

Table 7.1 Actions of angiotensin II via AT_1 and AT_2 receptor stimulation

AT_1 receptor stimulation
  Vasoconstriction (preferentially coronary, renal, cerebral)
  Steroidogenic (aldosterone)
  Dipsogenic (central nervous system effect)
  Renin suppression (negative feedback)
  Trophic and mitogenic (cardiac and vascular myocytes)
  Inotropic and contractile (cardiomyocytes)
  Chronotropic and arythmogenic (cardiomyocytes)
  Thrombogenic (plasminogen activator inhibitor)
  Oxidative (generation of reactive oxygen species)
  Ion transport channels (myocytes, renal cells)
  Neuroexcitation (sympathetic nerve terminals)
  Endothelin stimulation (endothelial cells)

AT_2 receptor stimulation
  Antiproliferation and inhibition of cell growth
  Cell differentiation
  Tissue repair
  Vasodilation
  Apoptosis

conditions in which the expression of AT_2 receptors is up-regulated, and AT_2 receptors may sometimes have a functional role in counterbalancing effects of AT_1 receptors (e.g. growth stimulation).[4–6] There are also recent experimental data suggesting that AT_2 receptor stimulation can trigger release of bradykinin, nitric oxide, and cyclic GMP release. Nevertheless, whether AT_2 receptors play a role in human cardiovascular homeostasis remains largely unknown.

ACE inhibition and AT_1 receptor blockade: are there theoretical differences?

As shown in *Fig. 7.1*, three groups of drugs have been developed to block the system at different sites (i.e. renin inhibitors, ACE inhibitors and angiotensin II receptor antagonists). Because ACE inhibitors and angiotensin II blockers act on different targets, potential differences between them may be expected, at least theoretically.

ACE inhibition blocks angiotensin I and bradykinin breakdown and metabolization of other peptides such as substance P. These peptides are without any doubt the source of the most common side effects of ACE inhibitors (cough, exaggerated allergic reactions, and, in rare cases, angioedema). However, there is limited evidence to suggest that the accumulation of bradykinin and other non-angiotensin peptides contributes to the beneficial effects of ACE inhibitors, but this topic remains a matter of debate. It was proposed recently that some of the desirable effects of ACE inhibitors on systemic and renal hemodynamics could be reversed with the administration of a bradykinin antagonist.[9] Unfortunately, the effects of the bradykinin antagonist *per se* were not investigated. Furthermore, the bradykinin antagonist was not studied in combination with the angiotensin II antagonists and the investigators did not take into account the differences in pharmacokinetics between losartan and captopril. Thus, these data do not allow firm conclusions to be drawn on the role of bradykinin. Additional convincing evidence will have to be provided to support the hypothesis that bradykinin contributes to the antihypertensive efficacy and to the organ-protective effects of ACE inhibitors.

At peak, acute inhibition of ACE lowers plasma angiotensin II levels to almost undetectable levels.[10,11] However, this is not the case during chronic ACE inhibition. Indeed, although blood pressure is reduced throughout the day with the repeated administration of an ACE inhibitor, plasma angiotensin II levels are still measurable, though they are reduced at peak. The lack of complete disappearance of angiotensin II from plasma during chronic treatment has been explained in several ways. Plasma renin activity and plasma angiotensin I levels increase markedly during ACE inhibition. Since ACE activity is never totally inhibited around the clock with ACE inhibitors, even a small percentage of enzyme activity does lead to the generation of angiotensin II if the substrate (i.e. angiotensin I) is available in large amounts.[12]

Alternatively, it has been postulated that during chronic ACE inhibition, angiotensin II may be formed by other enzymatic pathways.[3,13] The reappearance of circulating angiotensin II is usually not associated with an increase in blood pressure, indicating that clinically there is no escape phenomenon with ACE inhibitors.[14] However, the persistence of measurable circulating angiotensin II in plasma suggests that the system is not always entirely blocked with ACE inhibitors, particularly at trough.

AT_1 receptor antagonists interfere more specifically with the renin–angiotensin system than ACE inhibitors. Thus, in contrast to ACE inhibitors, angiotensin II blockers do not produce any measurable accumulation of bradykinin. With the administration of angiotensin II antagonists, all the angiotensin II effects mediated by AT_1 receptors are blocked. Because the negative feedback on renin secretion is also interrupted, angiotensin II receptor blockade is associated with a marked accumulation of angiotensin II in the plasma. The high angiotensin II levels could lead to the stimulation of the unopposed AT_2 receptors and hypothetically provide additional benefits if AT_2 receptors have indeed a function in inhibiting growth. However, at the present time it is unclear whether the unopposed effects of angiotensin II on other binding sites are of any clinical significance to the cardiovascular effects and safety profile of angiotensin II receptor antagonists.

In summary, the main differences between ACE inhibitors and angiotensin II blockers, based only on their mechanisms of action, reside in their ability to stimulate AT_2 receptors and to interfere with bradykinin metabolism. To determine whether the specific blockade of AT_1 receptors will provide any advantage over ACE inhibitors other than avoiding the bradykinin-mediated side effects, the role of AT_2 receptors and the possible consequences of their long-term stimulation will have to be clarified in humans. In addition, it is crucial to elucidate the real contribution of bradykinin in mediating any of the beneficial effects of ACE inhibitors.

Comparative antihypertensive efficacy: ACE inhibition versus AT_1 receptor blockade

The antihypertensive efficacy of angiotensin II blockers has been investigated abundantly in recent years and several studies have demonstrated their efficacy in mild, moderate and severe hypertension. Losartan, valsartan, irbesartan, candesartan, telmisartan, and eprosartan lower blood pressure effectively in all hypertensive patients regardless of age, sex, and race.[15–20] Most antagonists appear to have a sustained antihypertensive effect at 24 hours, indicating their ability to be prescribed once daily.

Because they act on the same hormonal system, ACE inhibitors and angiotensin II blockers were often compared in controlled, parallel group studies of between 8 and 12 weeks' duration that included large numbers of patients with essential hypertension. In accordance with the lack of clear evidence supporting a strong bradykinin role in the sustained antihypertensive efficacy of ACE inhibitors, angiotensin II receptor antagonists were as effective as ACE inhibitors but had a better tolerability profile. Thus, studies conducted with losartan, valsartan, irbesartan, candesartan, and telmisartan have displayed similar antihypertensive efficacy in terms of blood pressure reduction at trough when compared with ACE inhibitors such as enalapril or lisinopril.[21–25] Occasionally, a greater fall in blood pressure was found with the ACE inhibitor,[26] but sometimes the angiotensin II antagonist was found to be more effective.[27,28] *Fig. 7.2* summarizes the results of several comparative studies conducted with the first four angiotensin II blockers that were available for such studies; enalapril was the control ACE inhibitor.

Comparative tolerability: ACE inhibition versus AT_1 receptor blockade

The main characteristic of angiotensin II receptor antagonists is their excellent tolerability profile, with an adverse event rate generally similar

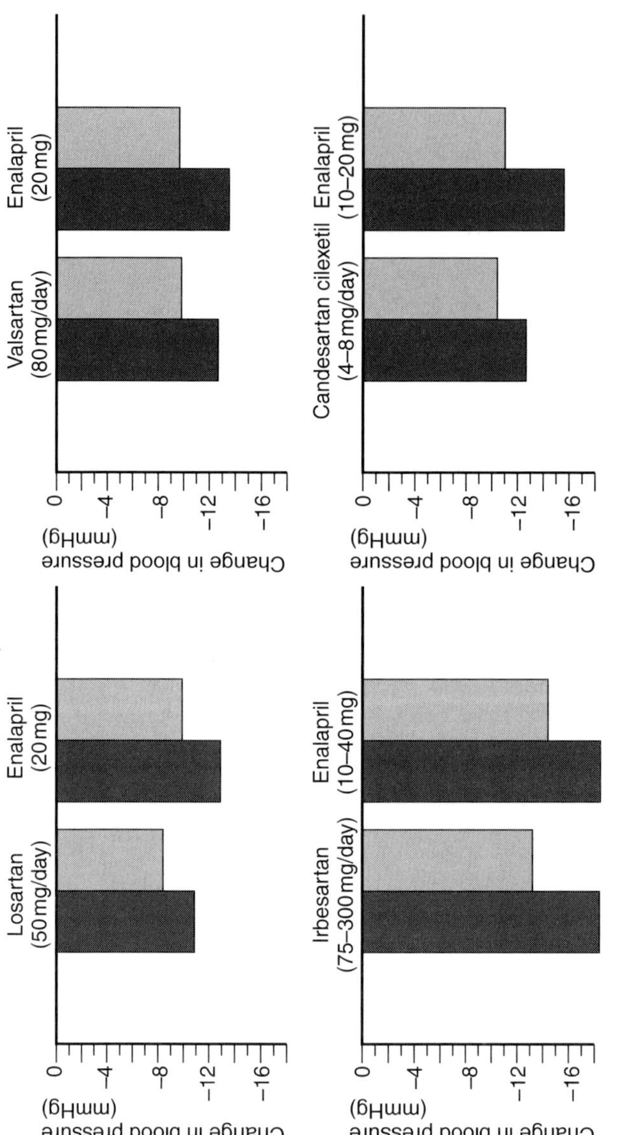

Figure 7.2

Changes in blood pressure induced by various angiotensin II receptor antagonists and enalapril in double-blind comparative studies conducted in mild-to-moderate hypertensive patients. Adapted from Chiolero and Burnier,[16] Tikkanen et al.,[21] Mimran et al.,[23] and Zanchetti et al.[24]

to placebo.[29] Cough is the most common side effect associated with the use of ACE inhibitors, with an incidence estimated at 5–20%. The development of angiotensin II blockers has provided an alternative to ACE inhibitors when blockade of the renin–angiotensin system is effective. Indeed, the administration of angiotensin II blockers has not been associated clinically with an increased occurrence of cough. Thus, the results of several large clinical trials have demonstrated that losartan causes a low level of spontaneous reports of cough in hypertensive patients (ranging from 2.3 to 4.1%).[30] This incidence was not different from placebo. The incidence of cough with candesartan, valsartan, and telmisartan was also comparable to that of the placebo groups.[11,31,32] In irbesartan-treated patients, cough was also less frequent than in patients receiving enalapril (10% versus 17%).[33]

Two double-blind studies have specifically addressed the issue of cough with patients complaining of cough while on ACE inhibitors.[34,35] In the first study, after a positive challenge with lisinopril, 135 patients were randomized in three parallel groups to receive lisinopril, losartan, or hydrochlorothiazide. After 8 weeks of treatment, the incidence of cough was comparable in the losartan and the hydrochlorothiazide groups and significantly lower than in the lisinopril group.[34] A similar study design was used to demonstrate that the occurrence of cough with valsartan is comparable to that observed with diuretic therapy but significantly lower than that observed with lisinopril.[35]

Angioedema is another adverse event associated with the use of ACE inhibitors. It occurs in about 0.1% of ACE inhibitor-treated patients.[36] The development of this side effect appears to involve the accumulation of bradykinin, but whether this is the only mechanism remains to be demonstrated.[36–38] To date, the data available do not allow to conclude firmly that angiotensin II receptor antagonists cause angioedema. Indeed, there are several reports in the literature of angioedema during losartan therapy, and several other cases may not have been reported.[39,40] Because angioedema can occur spontaneously or be triggered by many substances, including drugs and some foods, whether the reported episodes truly represent a specific side effect linked to angiotensin II receptor blockade is difficult to ascertain, but it seems rather unlikely.

Ageusia is a rare complication of ACE inhibitors that has been reported when higher doses of ACE inhibitors (mostly captopril) were used.[41] Two reports describe cases of patients with progressive dysgeusia or ageusia on treatment with losartan that were reversed after withdrawal of the drug.[42,43]

In general, angiotensin II blockers are neutral with regard to metabolic parameters. Whether angiotensin II antagonists improve insulin sensitivity as demonstrated with ACE inhibitors is still unclear.[44–46] Indeed, insulin sensitivity was not affected by a long-term administration of losartan whereas it was improved significantly with the use of candesartan.[45,46]

In post-transplant erythrocytosis, ACE inhibitors have been shown to suppress erythropoiesis. Several case reports and studies in renal transplant patients have suggested that losartan can also lower hematocrit effectively in this situation.[47–51] These results would seem to indicate that the stimulating effect that angiotensin II has on erythrocytosis in post-transplant patients might be due to the stimulation of AT_1 receptors.

Comparative renal and cardiac effects: ACE inhibition versus AT_1 receptor blockade

The renin–angiotensin system is an important component in the regulation of blood pressure and a crucial pathological factor in several models of renal dysfunction, ischemic heart disease, and heart failure. Hence, pharmacological interruption of the renin–angiotensin system with ACE inhibitors is now advocated as a standard therapeutic intervention for patients with chronic renal diseases and congestive heart failure. Do angiotensin II receptor blockers have a similar impact or a different one on renal hemodynamic and cardiac function?

Renal effects

The results obtained so far in experimental and clinical studies suggest that ACE inhibitors and angiotensin II receptor antagonists have similar effects on the kidney.[52–55] Indeed, several studies have demonstrated that angiotensin II antagonists have no effect on glomerular filtration and increase renal blood flow. This renal hemodynamic response to angiotensin II receptor blockade has been found in normotensive subjects[52,53] as well as in hypertensive patients.[54,55] Angiotensin II antagonists also increase urinary sodium excretion.[52,53] It has been postulated that the inhibition of prostaglandin metabolism is responsible for the ACE inhibitor-induced natriuresis. In a recent study, indomethacin has been found to abolish the natriuretic response to both ACE inhibition and angiotensin II receptor blockade in normotensive subjects.[56] This suggests that the antinatriuretic effect of non-steroidal anti-inflammatory drugs (NSAIDs) is not class-specific. Thus, one could expect clinically that NSAIDs blunt the antihypertensive effect of angiotensin II antagonists as they do with ACE inhibitors and diuretics. In a small group of 10 hypertensive patients, the administration of indomethacin did not attenuate the antihypertensive effect of losartan, although indomethacin significantly increased weight and promoted sodium retention.[57]

ACE inhibitors are also known to have a favorable impact on renal function because they reduce proteinuria. Several preliminary experimental and clinical studies involving small groups of patients have suggested that angiotensin II receptor antagonists have the same capacity to lower urinary albumin excretion as ACE inhibitors.[54] In a group of 20 patients with IgA nephropathy, both enalapril (20 mg/day) and irbesartan (100 mg/day) have been shown to reduce transglomerular passage of large test macromolecules without affecting the sieving coefficients of small dextran molecules.[58] This resulted in comparable decreases in urinary protein excretion.[58] Similar results were obtained with valsartan.[59] Furthermore, the antiproteinuric effect of angiotensin II receptor blockade appears to be potentiated by the administration of indomethacin in patients with human IgA nephropathy.[60]

Deterioration of renal function is a recognized side-effect of ACE inhibitors in patients with atheromatous bilateral renal artery stenosis, stenosis of a single functioning kidney, and unilateral stenosis associated with a contralateral nephrosclerosis. The fall in intraglomerular pressure that is caused by a decrease in efferent glomerular arteriole tone is considered to be the main mechanism leading to the ACE inhibitor-induced fall in glomerular filtration rate. However, some experimental data have suggested that the accumulation of endogenous kinins caused by ACE inhibition contributes to the deterioration of renal function in renal artery stenosis. In one double-blind, cross-over study involving 12 patients with unilateral renovascular disease, no change in renal function was observed after 4 days of treatment with valsartan (80 mg/day).[61] However, in another study that investigated 17 patients with atheromatous renal artery stenosis, single doses of captopril (50 mg) and losartan (200 mg) induced similar decreases in blood pressure and glomerular filtration rate.[62] Several other case reports have suggested that angiotensin II blockers can sometimes worsen renal function in renovascular disease.[63–66] Taken together, these preliminary results suggest that acute renal failure may occur with angiotensin II receptor antagonists, as it does with ACE inhibitors, when they are administered to patients with severe renal artery stenosis or diffuse intrarenal vascular sclerosis.

Deterioration of renal function is also a frequent complication in patients with severe heart failure treated with an ACE inhibitor. The primary end-point of the Evaluation of Losartan In the Elderly (ELITE) study was to compare the renal safety of captopril (50 mg q8h) and losartan (50 mg once daily) in elderly patients with heart failure by evaluating the proportion of patients who doubled their serum creatinine during treatment.[67] The results of this study show that the incidence of renal failure is similar with the two therapeutic approaches.

In contrast to all other angiotensin II blockers, losartan has been shown to increase urinary uric acid excretion and hence to lower plasma uric acid in normotensives.[52] The uricosuric effect of losartan is due to a specific effect of losartan on urate transport in the renal proximal tubule and is independent of angiotensin II receptor blockade.[68] EXP3174, the active metabolite of losartan, has no effect on uric acid excretion.[69] A decrease in serum uric acid levels has been found consistently in hypertensive patients treated with losartan. In diuretic-treated patients, the addition of losartan has been shown to prevent the diuretic-induced increase in serum uric acid.[70] The uricosuric effect of losartan is not associated with an increased incidence of urate stone formation. This may be due to the fact that losartan simultaneously increases urinary pH by decreasing the proximal reabsorption of bicarbonate.[52,71] In cyclosporine-treated hyperuricemic heart-transplant patients, losartan has also been shown to reduce serum uric acid levels.[72] The other non-peptide AT_1 antagonists have no effect on uric acid excretion.[53,73]

Cardiac effects

Regression of left ventricular hypertrophy is an important therapeutic goal in the treatment of hypertensive patients. Drugs such as ACE inhibitors have been shown to induce regression of left ventricular hypertrophy, and it has been suggested that, for a given fall in arterial pressure, the reduction in left ventricular mass is slightly more pronounced with ACE inhibitors than with conventional antihypertensive therapy.[74] Experimentally, angiotensin II blockers have been shown to induce left ventricular hypertrophy regression in hypertensive animals.[75] Clinically, there is also accumulating evidence to suggest that angiotensin II receptor blockade is associated with a reduction of left ventricular mass in hypertensive patients. In a comparative study, losartan had a greater effect on left ventricular mass than verapamil and hydrochlorothiazide.[76] In another study, a greater decrease in left ventricular mass index was found with valsartan (80–160 mg daily) than with atenolol (50–100 mg daily) in 58 patients with essential hypertension.[77] These results suggest that blockade of the renin–angiotensin system with angiotensin II blockers can induce regression of left ventricular mass. Whether this is due only to lowering blood pressure or also to interfering with the proliferative effect of angiotensin II is not clear yet.

In many countries, ACE inhibitors are recommended as first-line treatment for left ventricular systolic dysfunction, an indication in which ACE inhibitors have been shown to improve physical activity and reduce morbidity and mortality. ACE inhibitors are also recommended for all patients with heart failure who need treatment with diuretics. Several short-term studies conducted in patients with heart failure indicate that angiotensin II blockers are well tolerated and produce beneficial hemodynamic effects comparable to those of ACE inhibitors.[78–81] In the ELITE trial, patients treated with losartan (50 mg daily) were found to have a significantly lower rate of all-cause mortality and all-cause hospitalization than those receiving captopril 50 mg q8h.[67] However, these results were not confirmed by the recently presented ELITE II study. Since this latter study was not powered to demonstrate an equivalence between the drugs, one cannot ascertain that captopril (50 mg q8h) and losartan (50 mg daily) are equivalent. The potential benefits of angiotensin II blockers in heart failure have also been questioned by the premature interruption of the RESOLVD trial, in which 769 patients with symptomatic heart failure were randomized into six arms: candesartan alone in three different doses (4 mg daily, 8 mg daily, 16 mg daily), a combination of candesartan in two doses (4 mg daily and 8 mg daily) plus enalapril (10 mg q12hr) or enalapril alone (10 mg q12hr).[82] The preliminary results of this study suggested that there was a greater number of cardiovascular deaths among patients receiving candesartan (either alone or in combination) than there was among those treated with enalapril alone. However, the differences were not statistically significant. It is therefore impossible to draw conclusions from these results and it would be premature to conclude that angiotensin II receptor blockade causes any harm in patients with heart failure. The results of the ELITE II and the RESOLVD trials further emphasizes the need for larger mortality trials with angiotensin II blockers in heart failure.

Angiotensin II blockers and ACE inhibitors: a useful combination?

If there is concern about incomplete blockade of the renin–angiotensin system with ACE inhibitors, additional efficacy could be expected, at least theoretically, from the combination of an ACE inhibitor with an AT_1 receptor antagonist, because the antagonist blocks angiotensin II independently of its source. However, if the antagonist effectively blocks all the effects of angiotensin II independently of the level of circulating angiotensin II, the need for an ACE inhibitor would be doubtful. Plasma angiotensin II levels increase markedly during chronic blockade of AT_1 receptors. The elevated plasma angiotensin II levels can be expected to compete with the antagonist at the receptor site and to displace the antagonist from the receptor. In this situation, the added ACE inhibitor could blunt the rise in plasma angiotensin II and thereby increase the antihypertensive efficacy of the receptor antagonist. Whether this hypothesis holds true in clinical hypertension and, more precisely, whether high circulating angiotensin II levels are indeed able to compete with the mostly insurmountable receptor blockade certainly deserves further investigation. A blunting of the reactive rise in circulating angiotensin II could also potentially decrease the efficacy of the angiotensin II blockers by causing less AT_2 receptor stimulation. In any case, a combined therapy will certainly not avoid the side effects of ACE inhibition.

Several investigators have explored the potential benefits of a combination of ACE inhibitors and angiotensin II blockers in various clinical conditions. In salt-depleted normotensive volunteers, the combined administration of a standard single oral dose of an ACE inhibitor (captopril 50 mg) and an angiotensin II antagonist (losartan 50 mg) has been shown to induce an additional blood pressure reduction characterized mainly by a longer duration, and to have a major additive effect on the reactive rise in plasma renin activity.[83] Based on this result, it was proposed that a combination of an ACE inhibitor with an AT_1 receptor antagonist could achieve a more complete blockade of the renin–angiotensin system than either therapeutic approach alone. However, it was shown recently that all antagonists do not provide the same degree of angiotensin II receptor blockade, at least at the recommended starting dose, and that a greater reactive rise in plasma angiotensin II levels can be obtained with 150 mg irbesartan than with 50 mg losartan.[84] Thus, a more complete blockade could possibly be achieved with a greater dose of an AT_1 receptor antagonist alone.

Several studies have been conducted in renal diseases and heart failure to evaluate the interest of an ACE inhibitor–AT_1 receptor antagonist combination. Thus, in rats that had had five-sixths of their renal tissue ablated, enalapril, losartan, and the combination of both agents had similar renoprotective effects.[85] The renal protection was closely related to the magnitude of the antihypertensive effects. This observation suggests that there is no advantage in the combination of an ACE inhibitor and an angiotensin II receptor antagonists that goes beyond blood pressure control. In contrast to these data, the addition of an angiotensin blocker to ACE inhibitor therapy appeared to produce more profound decreases in proteinuria in hypertensive patients with diabetic nephropathy and in normotensive patients with IgA nephropathy and proteinuria.[86,87] However, these observations were gathered on a relatively small number of patients, and high doses of the angiotensin II antagonists were not investigated. Therefore, they deserve confirmation on larger groups of patients.

In congestive heart failure, high doses of ACE inhibitors are often necessary to block the renin–angiotensin system. In this condition, the association of an ACE inhibitor and an AT_1 receptor antagonist could seem attractive to improve the overall blockade of the system.[88–91] Preliminary studies have shown that a combination of losartan and enalapril was well tolerated in patients with heart failure and that the combined therapy resulted in greater effect than enalapril alone in terms of suppression of aldosterone and norepinephrine.[88] Similar results were reported recently with the use of valsartan.[89] In patients with anterior myocardial infarction, the combination of losartan (25 mg daily) and captopril (75 mg daily) was also well tolerated and more effective than captopril alone.[91] Again, full dosing ranges of the AT_1 receptor blockers were hardly explored.

In summary, additional large clinical trials are definitively needed to decide whether the combination of an ACE inhibitor with an AT_1 receptor antagonist provides additive—or even synergistic—therapeutic benefits in patients with hypertension, heart failure, or diabetic nephropathy.

Table 7.2 Summary of ongoing clinical trials with angiotensin II blockers

Angiotensin II blocker	Trial	Population	End-point	Completion
Losartan	ELITE II	Heart failure	All-cause mortality	1999
	LIFE	Hypertensives with left ventricular hypertrophy	Mortality, myocardial infarction, stroke	2001
	OPTIMAAL	Post-myocardial infarction with left ventricular dysfunction	All cause mortality	2000
	RENAAL	Non-insulin-dependent diabetes mellitus patients with nephropathy	Composite of ESRD, doubling of creatinine, mortality	2001
Valsartan	Val-HeFT	Heart failure	All-cause mortality	2001
	VALIANT	Post-myocardial infarction with left ventricular dysfunction	All-cause mortality	2005
	VALUE	Hypertensives with high risk	Cardiovascular mortality	2004
	ABCD-2C	Non-insulin dependent diabetes mellitus patients	Composite of end-stage renal disease, doubling of creatinine, mortality	2003
Candesartan	CHARM I	Heart failure, ACE inhibitor-intolerant	All-cause mortality	2002
	CHARM II	Heart failure	All-cause mortality	2002
	CHARM III	Heart failure (left ventricular ejection fraction > 0.40)	All-cause mortality	2002
	SCOPE	Elderly hypertensives	Cardiovascular mortality, myocardial infarction, stroke	2001
Irbesartan	IDNT	Non-insulin-dependent diabetes mellitus patients with nephropathy	Composite of end-stage renal disease, doubling of creatinine, mortality	2000

However, to demonstrate the advantages of an ACE-inhibitor–AT_1 antagonist combination, this combination should be compared clinically with a full titration of each individual drug using also long-acting angiotensin II antagonists. *A priori* it seems highly questionable to attempt complete blockade of the renin–angiotensin system by a combination of an ACE inhibitor and an AT_1 receptor antagonist if the same result could be achieved by a higher dose of an AT_1 receptor antagonist alone (without adding the side effects inherent to all ACE inhibitors).

Comparisons of angiotensin II blockers and ACE inhibitors in large ongoing trials

Several large clinical trials are currently underway with the various angiotensin II antagonists. These trials seek to establish the morbidity and mortality benefits of specific AT_1 receptor blockade in patients with hypertension (with or without left ventricular hypertrophy), heart failure, acute myocardial infarction, and non-insulin-dependent diabetic nephropathy (*Table 7.2*). Several questions about the use of angiotensin II blockers should be resolved by these studies. In particular, they will help to determine whether the mechanistic differences between ACE inhibitors and angiotensin II blockers lead to significant clinical differences. Moreover, they will provide further information on the potential benefits of the combination of ACE inhibitors and angiotensin II blockers.

Unfortunately, angiotensin II receptor antagonists and ACE inhibitors will not be compared for their ability to prevent diabetic or non-diabetic nephropathies or to promote left ventricular mass regression in hypertensive patients. However, the morbidity and mortality benefits of angiotensin II blockers alone or in combination with ACE inhibitors will be assessed in patients with heart failure. Thus, ELITE II, Val-HeFT[92] and the CHARM studies are complementary trials which will provide more insight in the potential of angiotensin II receptor blockade in heart failure.[93] They will also address several practical issues such as dosing (once versus twice daily, monotherapy versus combination) and the efficacy in different populations (ACE inhibitor-naïve patients, ACE inhibitor-intolerant patients, and patients with diastolic dysfunction). Two studies, the OPTI-MAAL trial[94] and the VALIANT trials, will be conducted in post-myocardial infarction.[93] In both cases, the effects of the angiotensin blocker (losartan in OPTIMAAL and valsartan in VALIANT) will be compared to captopril. In OPTIMAAL, losartan is given once daily as monotherapy whereas in VALIANT, valsartan is given twice daily and in combination with an ACE inhibitor. Again, the results of these two trials will establish whether combination therapy is useful for optimum clinical effect. They may also provide additional information on the role of bradykinin and AT_2 receptors in the effects of angiotensin II blockers and ACE inhibitors.

Conclusions

Taken together, the clinical data presented in this chapter demonstrate that angiotensin II receptor blockers have a similar antihypertensive efficacy to that of ACE inhibitors but a better tolerability profile. Thus, for the treatment of essential hypertension, angiotensin II blockers will probably replace ACE inhibitors in time unless the large clinical trials demonstrate unexpected harmful effects or a surprising lack of improvement in morbidity and mortality.

Whether angiotensin II blockers should be added on an ACE inhibitor therapy definitely deserves further investigations. We do not yet have enough information from well-designed studies to support a clear benefit of the combination. Additional trials should be conducted in diseases such as diabetic and non-diabetic nephropathy to investigate the potential benefits of the combination on proteinuria and the progression of renal disease. However, these investigations should include the exploration of full dosing ranges of the AT_1 receptor blockers given alone. The ongoing trials in heart failure and left ventricular dysfunction post-myocardial infarction will elucidate whether there is any clinical advantage in using angiotensin II blockers alone or in combination with ACE inhibitors in these indications.

References

1. Houghton AR, Cowley AJ. Why are angiotensin converting enzyme inhibitors underutilised in the treatment of heart failure by general practitioners? Int J Cardiol 1997; 59: 7–10.

2. Timmermans PBMWM, Wong PC, Chiu AT *et al*. Angiotensin II receptors and angiotensin II receptor antagonists. Pharmacol Review 1993; 45: 205–251.

3. Dzau VJ, Sasamura H, Hein L. Heterogeneity of angiotensin synthetic pathways and receptor subtypes: physiological and pharmacological implications. J Hypertens 1993; 11 (suppl 11): S13–S18.

4. Stoll M, Steckelings UM, Paul M *et al*. The angiotensin AT_2-receptor mediates inhibition of cell proliferation in coronary endothelial cells. J Clin Invest 1995; 95: 651–657.

5. Meffert S, Stoll M, Steckelings UM *et al*. The angiotensin II AT_2 receptor inhibits proliferation and promotes differentiation in Pc12W cells. Moll Cell Endocrinol 1996; 1222: 59–67.

6. Ohkubo N, Matsubara H, Nozawa Y *et al*. Angiotensin type 2 receptors are re-expressed by cardiac fibroblasts from failing myopathic hamster hearts and inhibit cell growth and fibrillar collagen metabolism. Circulation 1997; 96: 3954–3962.

7. Gohlke P, Pees C, Unger T. AT_2 receptor stimulation increases aortic cyclic GMP in SHRSP by a kinin-dependent mechanism. Hypertension 1998; 31: 349–355.

8. Siragy HM, Inagami T, Carey RM. Sustained hypersensitivity of angiotensin II and its mechanism in mice lacking the subtype-2

(AT$_2$) angiotensin receptor. Proc Natl Acad Sci USA 1999; in press.

9. Gainer JV, Morrow JD, Loveland AL *et al.* Effect of bradykinin-receptor blockade on the response to angiotensin-converting-enzyme inhibitor in normotensive and hypertensive subjects. N Eng J Med 1998; 339: 1285–1292.

10. Nussbeger J, Waeber B, Brunner HR. Clinical pharmacology of ACE inhibition. Cardiology 1989; 76 (suppl 2): 11–22.

11. Nussberger J, Brunner DB, Waeber B, Brunner HR. True versus immunoreactive angiotensin II in human plasma. Hypertension 1985; 7 (suppl I): I1–I7.

12. Mooser V, Nussberger J, Juillerat L *et al.* Reactive hyperreninemia is a major determinant of plasma angiotensin II during ACE inhibition. J Cardiovasc Pharmacol 1990; 15: 276–282.

13. Urata K, Kinoshita A, Misono K *et al.* Identification of a highly specific chymase as the major angiotensin-forming enzyme in the human heart. J Biol Chem 1990; 265: 22348–22382.

14. Brunner HR, Gavras H, Waeber B *et al.* Oral angiotensin-converting enzyme inhibitor in long-term treatment of hypertensive patients. Ann Intern Med 1979; 90: 19–23.

15. Johnston CI. Angiotensin receptor antagonist: focus on losartan. Lancet 1995; 346: 1403–1407.

16. Chiolero A, Burnier M. Pharmacology of valsartan, an angiotensin II receptor antagonist. Expert Opin Investig Drugs 1998; 7: 1915–1925.

17. Reeves RA, Lin CS, Kassler-Taub K, Pouleur H. Dose-related efficacy of irbesartan for hypertension. An integrated analysis. Hypertension 1998; 31: 1311–1316.

18. Sever P. Candesartan cilexetil: a new, long-acting, effective angiotensin II type 1 receptor blocker. J Human Hypertens 1997; 11 (suppl 2): S91–S95.

19. McClellan KJ, Markham A. Telmisartan. Drugs 1998; 56: 1039–1044.

20. McClellan KJ, Balfour JA. Eprosartan. Drugs 1998; 55: 713–718.

21. Tikkanen I, Omvik P, Jensen HA for the Scandinavian Study Group. Comparison of the angiotensin II antagonist losartan with the angiotensin converting enzyme inhibitor enalapril in patients with essential hypertension. J Hypertens 1995; 13: 1343–1351.

22. Black HR, Graff A, Shute D *et al.* Valsartan, a new angiotensin II antagonist for the treatment of essential hypertension: efficacy, tolerability and safety compared to an angiotensin-converting enzyme inhibitor, lisinopril. J Hum Hypertens 1997; 11: 483–489.

23. Mimran A, Ruilope L, Kerwin L *et al.* A randomised, double-blind comparison of the angiotensin II receptor antagonist, irbesartan, with the full dose range of enalapril for the treatment of mild-to-moderate hypertension. J Hum Hypertens 1998; 12: 203–208.

24. Zanchetti A, Omboni S, DiBaggio C, on behalf of the Study Group. Candesartan cilexetil and enalapril are of equivalent efficacy in patients with mild to moderate hypertension. J Hum Hypertens 1997; 11 (suppl 2): S57–S59.

25. Neutel J, Frishman W, Oparil S *et al.* A comparison of telmisartan with lisinopril in patients with mild to moderate hypertension (abstract). Am J Hypertens 1998; 1: 115A.

26. Gradman AH, Arcuri KE, Gold-

berg AI *et al.* A randomized, placebo-controlled, double-blind, parallel study of various doses of losartan potassium compared with enalapril maleate in patients with essential hypertension. Hypertension 1995; 25: 1345–1350.

27. Smith DHG, Neutel JM, Morgenstern P. Once-daily telmisartan compared with enalapril in the treatment of hypertension. Adv Ther 1998; 15: 229–240.

28. Ponticelli C, the Eprosartan Study Group. Comparison of the efficacy of eprosartan and enalapril in patients with severe hypertension (abstract). Am J Hypertens 1997; 10: 128A.

29. Mazzolai L, Burnier M. Comparative safety and tolerability of angiotensin II receptor antagonists. Drug Saf 1999; 21: 23–33.

30. Lacourcière Y, Lefebvre J, Nakhle G *et al.* Association between cough and angiotensin converting enzyme inhibitory versus angiotensin II antagonists: the design of a prospective, controlled study. J Hypertens 1994; 12: 549–553.

31. Belcher G, Hübner R, George M *et al.* Candesartan cilexetil: safety and tolerability in healthy volunteers and patients with hypertension. J Hum Hypertens 1998; 11: S85–S89.

32. Neutel JM. Safety and efficacy of angiotensin II receptor antagonists. Am J Cardiol 1999; 84: (suppl 2) 13K–17K.

33. Gillis JC, Markham A. Irbesartan: a review of its pharmacodynamic and pharmacokinetic properties and therapeutic use in the management of hypertension. Drugs 1997; 54: 885–902.

34. Lacourcière Y, Brunner HR, Irwing R *et al.* Effects of modulators of the renin–angiotensin–aldosterone system on cough. J Hypertens 1994; 12: 1387–1393.

35. Benz J, Oshrain C, Henry D *et al.* Valsartan, a new angiotensin II receptor antagonist: a double-blind study comparing the incidence of cough with lisinopril and hydrochlorothiazide. J Clin Pharmacol 1997; 37: 101–107.

36. Israili ZH, Hall WD. Cough and angioneurotic edema associated with angiotensin-converting enzyme inhibitor therapy. A review of the literature and pathophysiology. Ann Intern Med 1992; 117: 234–242.

37. Nussberger J, Cugno M, Amstutz C *et al.* Plasma bradykinin in angio-oedema. Lancet 1998; 351: 1693–1697.

38. Vleeming W, van Amsterdam JG, Stricker BH, de Wildt DJ. ACE inhibitor-induced angioedema. Incidence, prevention and management. Drug Saf 1998; 18: 171–188.

39. Acker G, Greenberg A. Angioedema induced by the angiotensin II blocker losartan. N Engl J Med 1995; 333: 1572.

40. van Rijnsoever EW, Kwee-Zuiderwijk WJ, Feenstra J. Angioneurotic edema attributed to the use of losartan. Arch Intern Med 1998; 158: 2063–2065.

41. Griffin J. Drug-induced disorders of taste. Adverse Drug React Toxicol 1992; 11: 229–239.

42. Schlienger R, Saxer M, Haefli W. Reversible ageusia associated with losartan. Lancet 1996; 347: 471–472.

43. Heeringa M, van Puijenbroek EP. Reversible dysgeusia attributed to losartan. Ann Intern Med 1998; 129: 72.

44. Moan A, Hoieggen A, Seljeflot I *et al.* The effect of angiotensin II receptor antagonism with losartan on glucose metabolism and insulin sensitivity. J Hypertens 1996; 14: 1093–1097.

45. Laakso M, Karjalainen L, Lempiäinen-Kuosa P. Effects of losartan on insulin sensitivity in hypertensive subjects. Hypertension 1996; 28: 392–396.

46. Iimura O, Shimamoto K, Matsuda K *et al.* Effects of angiotensin receptor antagonist and angiotensin converting enzyme inhibitor on insulin sensitivity in fructose-fed rats and essential hypertensives. Am J Hypertens 1995; 8: 353–357.

47. Julian BA, Brantley RR Jr, Barker CV *et al.* Losartan, an angiotensin II type 1 receptor antagonist, lowers hematocrit in posttransplant erythrocytosis. J Am Soc Nephrol 1998; 9: 1104–1108.

48. Schwarzbeck A, Wittenmeier KW, Hallfritzsch U. Anaemia in dialysis patients as a side-effect of sartanes. Lancet 1998; 352: 286.

49. Navarro JF, Garcia J, Macia M *et al.* Effects of losartan on the treatment of posttransplant erythrocytosis. Clin Nephrol 1998; 49: 370–372.

50. Ducloux D, Fournier V, Bresson-Vautrin C, Chalopin JM. Long-term follow-up of renal transplant recipients treated with losartan for post-transplant erythrosis. Transpl Int 1998; 11: 312–315.

51. Hortal L, Fernandez A, Vega N *et al.* Losartan versus ramipril in the treatment of postrenal transplant erythrocytosis. Transpl Proc 1998; 30: 2127–2128.

52. Burnier M, Rutschmann B, Nussberger J *et al.* Salt-dependent renal effects of angiotensin II antagonist in healthy subjects. Hypertension 1993; 22: 339–347.

53. Burnier M, Hagman M, Nussberger J *et al.* Short-term and sustained renal effects of angiotensin II receptor blockade in healthy subjects. Hypertension 1995; 25: 602–609.

54. Gansevoort RT, DeZeeuw D, de Jong PE. Is the antiproteinuric effect of ACE inhibition mediated by interference in the renin–angiotensin system? Kidney Int 1994; 45: 861–867.

55. Pechère-Bertschi A, Nussberger J, Decosterd L *et al.* Renal response to the AT_1 antagonist irbesartan vs enalapril hypertensive patients. J Hypertens 1998; 16: 385–393.

56. Fricker A, Nussberger J, Meilenbrock S *et al.* Effect of indomethacin on the renal response to angiotensin II receptor blockade in healthy subjects. Kidney Int 1998; 54: 2089–2097.

57. Olsen ME, Thomsen T, Hassager C *et al.* Hemodynamic and renal effects of indomethacin in losartan-treated hypertensive individuals. Am J Hypertens 1999; 12: 209–216.

58. Remuzzi A, Perico N, Sangalli F *et al.* ACE inhibition and Ang II receptor blockade improve glomerular size-selectivity in IgA nephropathy. Am J Physiol 1999; 276: F457–F466.

59. Plum J, Buenten B, Nemeth R, Grabensee B. Effects of the angiotensin II antagonist valsartan on blood pressure, proteinuria, and renal hemodynamics in patients with chronic renal failure and hypertension. J Am Soc Nephrol 1998; 9: 2223–2234.

60. Perico N, Remuzzi A, Sangalli F *et al.* The antiproteinuric effect of angiotensin antagonism in human IgA nephropathy is potentiated by indomethacin. J Am Soc Nephrol 1998; 9: 2308–2317.

61. Arzilli F, Favilla S, Motolese M *et al.* Valsartan, a new angiotensin II antagonist: tolerability and effects on renal function in patients with renovascular arterial hypertension. High Blood Press 1997; 6: 153–158.

62. Mimran A, Ribstein J, DuCailar G. Comparison of the acute renal effect of losartan and captopril in atheromatous renovascular disease (abstract). Am J Hypertens 1998; 11: 47A.

63. Saine D, Ahrens E. Renal impairment associated with losartan. Ann Intern Med 1996; 124: 775.

64. Holm EA, Randlov A, Strandgard S. Acute renal failure after losartan treatment in a patient with bilateral renal artery stenosis. Blood Press 1996; 5: 360–362.

65. Missouris CG, Ward DE, Eastwood JB, MacGregor GA. Deterioration in renal function with enalapril but not losartan in a patient with renal artery stenosis in a solitary kidney. Heart 1997; 77: 391–392.

66. Ostermann M, Goldsmith DJA, Doyle T et al. Reversible acute renal failure induced by losartan in a renal transplant recipient. Postgrad Med J 1997; 73: 105–107.

67. Pitt B, Segal R, Martinez FA et al. Randomised trial of losartan versus captopril in patients over 65 with heart failure (Evaluation of Losartan In The Elderly study, ELITE). Lancet 1997; 349: 747–752.

68. Burnier M, Roch-Ramel F, Brunner HR. Renal effects of angiotensin II receptor blockade in normotensive subjects. Kidney Int 1996; 49: 1787–1790.

69. Sweet CS, Bradstreet DC. Berman RS et al. Pharmacodynamic activity of intravenous E-3174, an angiotensin II antagonist, in patients with essential hypertension. Am J Hypertens 1994; 7: 1035–1040.

70. Soffer BA, Wright JT, Pratt H et al. Effects of losartan on a background of hydrochlorothiazide in patients with hypertension. Hypertension 1995; 26: 112–117.

71. Shahinfar S, Simpson C, Carides A et al. Safety of losartan in hyper-tensive patients with asymptomatic hyperuricemia. J Am Soc Nephrol 1997; 8: 322A.

72. Minghelli G, Seydoux C, Goy J, Burnier M. Uricosuric effect of losartan in cyclosporine-treated heart transplant recipients. Transplantation 1998; 66: 268–271.

73. Ilson BE, Martin DE, Boike SC, Jorkasky DK. The effects of eprosartan, an angiotensin II AT1 receptor antagonist, on uric acid excretion in patients with mild to moderate essential hypertension. J Clin Pharmacol 1998; 38: 437–441.

74. Schmieder RE, Schlaich MP. Comparison of therapeutic studies on regression of left ventricular hypertrophy. Adv Exp Med Biol 1997; 432: 191–198.

75. Bohm M, Lee M, Kreuz R et al. Angiotensin II receptor blockade in TGR(mREN2)27: effects of renin–angiotensin system gene expression and cardiovascular functions. J Hypertens 1995; 13: 891–899.

76. Tedesco MA, Ratti G, Aquino D et al. Effects of losartan on hypertension and left ventricular mass: a long-term study. J Hum Hypertens 1998; 12: 505–510.

77. Thuermann PA, Kenedi P, Schmidt A et al. Influence of the angiotensin II antagonist valsartan on left ventricular hypertrophy in patients with essential hypertension. Circulation 1998; 98: 2037–2042.

78. Gottlieb SS, Dickstein K, Fleck E et al. Hemodynamic and neurohormonal effects of the angiotensin II antagonist losartan in patients with congestive heart failure. Circulation 1993; 8: 1602–1609.

79. Dickstein K, Chang P, Willenheimer R, Haunso S et al. Comparison of the effects of losartan and enalapril on clinical status and exercise performance in patients with moderate or severe heart

failure. J Am Coll Cardiol 1995; 26: 438–445.

80. Crozier I, Ikram H, Awan N *et al.* for the Losartan Hemodynamic Study Group. Losartan in heart failure. Hemodynamic effects and tolerability. Circulation 1995; 91: 691–697.

81. Havranek EP, Thomas I, Smith WB *et al.* Dose-related beneficial long term hemodynamic and clinical efficacy of irbesartan in heart failure. J Am Coll Cardiol 1999; 33: 1174–1181.

82. Anonymous. Phase I results of the randomized evaluation of left ventricular dysfunction (RESOLVD) trial. Am J Managed Care 1998; 4: S380–S383.

83. Azizi M, Chatellier G, Guyene TT *et al.* Additive effects of combined angiotensin-converting enzyme inhibition and angiotensin II antagonism on blood pressure and renin release in sodium-depleted normotensives. Circulation 1995; 92: 825–834.

84. Mazzolai L, Maillard M, Rossat J *et al.* Angiotensin II receptor blockade in normal subjects: a direct comparison of three AT_1 receptor antagonists. Hypertension 1999; 33: 850–855.

85. Ots M, MacKenzie HS, Troy JL *et al.* Effects of combination therapy with enalapril and losartan on the rate of progression of renal injury in rats with 5/6 renal mass ablation. J Am Soc Nephrol 1998; 9: 224–230.

86. Hebert LA, Falkenheim ME, Nahman NS *et al.* Combination ACE inhibitor and angiotensin II receptor antagonist therapy in diabetic nephropathy. Am J Nephrol 1999; 19: 1–6.

87. Russo D, Pisani A, Balletta MM *et al.* Additive antiproteinuric effect of converting enzyme inhibitor and losartan in normotensive patients with IgA nephropathy. Am J Kidney Dis 1999; 33: 851–856.

88. Pitt B, Dickstein K, Benedict C *et al.* Combined treatment with losartan and enalapril vs enalapril on neurohormonal activation in patients with heart failure (abstract). Circulation 1996; 94: I-428.

89. Baruch L, Anand I, Cohen IS *et al.* Augmented short- and long-term hemodynamic and hormonal effects of an angiotensin receptor blocker added to an angiotensin converting enzyme inhibitor therapy in patients with heart failure. Circulation 1999; 99: 2658–2664.

90. Hamroff G, Katz SD, Mancini D *et al.* Addition of angiotensin II receptor blockade to maximal angiotensin-converting enzyme inhibition improves exercise capacity in patients with severe congestive heart failure. Circulation 1999; 99: 990–992.

91. Di Pasquale P, Bucca V, Scalzo S, Paterna S. Safety, tolerability, and neurohormonal changes of the combination captopril plus losartan in the early post-infarction period: a pilot study. Cardiovasc Drugs Ther 1998; 12: 211–216.

92. Anonymous. Val-HeFT to investigate valsartan in treatment of congestive heart failure. Can J Cardiol 1997; 13: 971–972.

93. Willenheimer R, Dahlöf B, Rydberg E, Erhardt L. AT_1-receptor blockers in hypertension and heart failure: clinical experience and future directions. Eur Heart J 1999; 20: 997–1008.

94. Dickstein K, Kjekshus J for the OPTIMAAL Study Group. Comparison of the effects of losartan and captopril on mortality in patients following acute myocardial infarction. The OPTIMAAL trial design. Optimal Therapy In Myocardial infarction with the Angiotensin II Antagonist Losartan. Am J Cardiol 1999; 83: 477–481.

Index